Surface Tensions

To Mardi Manderson,
my mother, with love

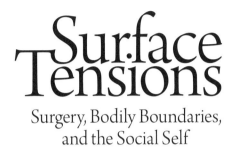

Surface Tensions

Surgery, Bodily Boundaries, and the Social Self

Lenore Manderson

Left Coast
Press Inc.

Walnut Creek, California

green press
INITIATIVE

Left Coast Press is committed to preserving ancient forests and natural resources. We elected to print this title on 30% post consumer recycled paper, processed chlorine free. As a result, for this printing, we have saved:

3 Trees (40' tall and 6-8" diameter)
1 Million BTUs of Total Energy
263 Pounds of Greenhouse Gases
1,185 Gallons of Wastewater
75 Pounds of Solid Waste

Left Coast Press made this paper choice because our printer, Thomson-Shore, Inc., is a member of Green Press Initiative, a nonprofit program dedicated to supporting authors, publishers, and suppliers in their efforts to reduce their use of fiber obtained from endangered forests.

For more information, visit www.greenpressinitiative.org

Environmental impact estimates were made using the Environmental Defense Paper Calculator. For more information visit: www.papercalculator.org.

Left Coast Press, Inc.
1630 North Main Street, #400
Walnut Creek, CA 94596
www.LCoastPress.com

ISBN 978-1-61132-097-8 hardcover
ISBN 978-1-61132-098-5 paperback
eISBN 978-1-61132-099-2

Manderson, Lenore.
 Surface tensions : surgery, bodily boundaries, and the social self / Lenore Manderson.
    p. cm.
 Summary: "Surface Tensions is an expansive, yet intimate study of how people remake themselves after catastrophic bodily change—the loss of limbs, the loss of function, the loss or replacement of organs. Against a sweeping cultural backdrop of art, popular culture, and the history of science and medicine, Manderson uses narrative epistemology based on in-depth interviews with over 300 individuals to show how they re-establish the coherence of their bodies, identities, and biographies. In addition to offering important new insights into the care, rehabilitation, and rehabituation of post-trauma patients, Manderson's work challenges conventional ideas about the nature of embodiment and is an important contribution to medical anthropology, disability studies, and cultural studies"—Provided by publisher.
 Includes bibliographical references.
 ISBN 978-1-61132-097-8 (hardback)—ISBN 978-1-61132-098-5 (pbk.)—ISBN 978-1-61132-099-2 (ebook)
 1. Human body—Social aspects. 2. Body image. 3. People with disabilities—Psychology. 4. Medical anthropology. I. Title.
 HM636.M33 2011
 305.9'08–dc23

                    2011022295

Printed in the United States of America
∞™ The paper used in this publication meets the minimum requirements of American National Standard for Information Sciences—Permanence of Paper for Printed Library Materials, ANSI/NISO Z39.48–1992.

Cover design by Hannah Jennings
Cover illustration: Julie Rrap, *Body Double*, 2007. Courtesy of the artist and Roslyn Oxley9 Gallery, Sydney, Australia

Contents

*My purpose is to tell of bodies that have been transformed
into shapes of a different kind.*

—Ovid, *Metamorphoses*, Book I

Preface 🖐

If I had to choose a body part that reflected how I saw myself, it would be my hands. My fingers are tensile, animated, loquacious: they talk, complementing the mobility of my face. I was surprised by a series of portraits of me in 1982, therefore; my face alone seemed too static, too pensive, to be me. On stage around the same time, I performed Beckett's *Not I* (Beckett 1973); playing against type, the staging conventions confined me only to my lips and voice to project the character. Stripped of my eyes and brows, glares and furrows, posture and demeanor, and my hands, I was left only with my mouth to work the text. Not I, indeed.

Hence the irony now, as I write, that I have little function in one hand. As this book took form, so did the metamorphosis of my left hand – the bad, the weak, the feminine, the evil (Hertz 1960 [1909]). In the early days, it lay largely passive, framed by a scaffolding of compound plastic and rubber, wire, fishing line and elastic bands, my arm trussed with Velcro, my fingers in slings, the whole a marionette, a suspended puppet relying on a false voice. The dynamic dorsal splint gave my hand prehensile strength; without it I was mute. On the other side, the good right hand, clawed back, subdued. Hands are for duets, not solos. The singular wellness of the right was an embarrassment, overcompensating for its twin. The giant white mantis praying preternaturally over my hand was only one of several props. Other splints gave me alternatives to meet various functional needs. A static volar splint, sculptured from the same materials of plastic epoxy and Velcro, gave my thumb a cubby-hole to rest from the motility provided by other splints. And my old, worn, torn, grubby, elastic and metal brace, the one I wore to sleep; this was the brace that, at the onset of the rupturing of a nerve, reduced pain through immobilization, and reduced the risk of my hand freezing in an ungainly hold.

A decade on, my left hand still has reduced function, but I have capitalized on this – it gave me an added vehicle through which to think of body change and embodied crisis. The early clumsy braces are stored away as mementos of the early days. My hand now sits lightly in a frame of aluminum, stainless steel and leather. The brace itself is a performance piece, eccentric and magnetic. It lives its own history in performance and film (Woodson 2007).

Academic folklore holds that women who research and write about pregnancy and childbirth conceive in the course of their project. My son and daughter were thus prefigured (Crouch and Manderson 1993). Many other writers have written autobiographically and from scholarly standpoints about ailments that they have experienced, their own health status stimulating their research and/or creativity. Anthropologists including Murphy (1987), Rapp (1999) and Becker (1997), and essayists and creative writers, famously including Sontag (1978), in North America, Europe, Australia and elsewhere, have sought meaning by writing about their confrontations with disease and encounters with medicine (1996). But while they write about ailments that they have experienced, there appear to be no corollaries with pregnancy – no study of cancer forecasting the disease of the author, no research on aneurysm anticipating a researcher's collapse, no description of multiple sclerosis rehearsing its embodiment. Until now: my research on dramatic loss of body function was the augury of my palsy. Were I to indulge in so fanciful an explanation for my own turn in health, I should be grateful, for in undertaking the interviews that are the empirical basis of this book, I have worked with people who experienced far greater losses than my own.

Even so, after four days of breathtaking pain in my arm and increasing numbness and weakness in my hand, my wrist and fingers were flaccid. As the pain abated, so did all strength. Wrist drop. I had turned into one of the people I was studying. Without plan, without will, I crossed from the world of the able-bodied, where I was positioned empathetically but innocently, into the world of the dis-abled. My arm was a constant reminder. I could trace the hard edges of the radius and ulna, fold the wasted flesh that cloaked them. Its flaccidity was with me when I woke in the morning; for months, daily, I checked it for an overnight miracle. It was there at night; again for some months, I spent fifteen minutes before sleep using electromagnetic stimulation to try to tease the nerves to grow and the muscle to be strong, stretching the wrist, swapping to a night-time wrist-brace to prevent contortion in my sleep. Dealing with a body with lack can be a fulltime job. Now I ignore it as much I can. Donning the brace is as habitual as putting on shoes.

Yet as I learned to embody and live with loss, I monitored its impact. Unable to control my wrist or lift my fingers or grip with strength, and without clever splints and braces, I discovered extraordinary numbers of impediments and impositions. I found it hard, sometimes impossible, to tie my shoe laces, cut food to cook, eat with a knife and fork, hand-wash clothes, wash my hair, floss my teeth, insert earrings, put on a bra, zip up pants, pull on pantyhose, apply underarm deodorant, shave my armpits, clip my nails, smooth them with an emery board, paint them, bite them. I couldn't pick my nose, scratch my body. And – the ultimate irony for an academic – I couldn't shuffle through paper; filing away and retrieving papers, grabbing a book from a shelf, the mechanics of using a dictionary, became physical chores. These were all, excepting for paper shuffling, matters of bodily maintenance. Other things I couldn't do came to me more slowly. I can't dance freely; my left arm flops and flays. I can't caress: my left hand sits as a dead weight against my partner's body or around a child's back. I cannot cup fresh water from a spring and drink from my hands. I cannot play a guitar or a piano, even in theory, save for a few concerti for one hand. I cannot shape a snowball. I can't swing from a trapeze. I can't row a boat. I can't climb rocks, or climb the precarious exciting mountain faces that I had only just learned to grip without fear and with enormous triumph. I can't lift weights. I had to learn to swim with a limp hand. I will never ski. I can't clap. I know the sound of one hand clapping.

It is now convention for an academic work to begin with autobiography. Sometimes this seems a pretension, but here, my body is insinuated. Four months after the onset of excruciating, almost impossible pain, I stepped onto an escalator of diagnostics and experiments in rehabilitation: hospitals for neurological tests to establish that only the radial nerve was involved; visits to a rehabilitation medicine center for physiotherapy, occupational therapy and orthopedic splints; hospitals again for magnetic resonance imaging. Then surgery to explore and eliminate nerve compression as the cause of the paralysis. I spun into the disempowered state of patienthood. I was not sick on admission, just anxious and feeling somewhat fraudulent. Awakening as I was wheeled from the recovery room to the lift, I was heartened: now I was legitimately prone and under medical care. The surgery was disappointing though: no compression of the radial nerve, but distension, thickening, translucency, edema, lumps and turns. I saw the photographs the next day, emailed to me as .jpg files, the twisted nerve lying on a bed of bright tissue. The nerve was framed thickly by yellow subcutaneous fat, and vanity prevented me, almost, from emailing the photographs to others. But not quite: I took glee in responding to enquiries of my health with a supreme postmodern gesture – the surgeon's eye of my exposed flesh. And patienthood continued: tomography, more medical resonance imaging, nerve conduction studies, prednisolone, intravenous immunoglobulin, physiotherapy (Manderson 2002).

The pain was short-lived. The adaptation to loss of function took longer, but it was a practical challenge. And making friends with the brace was a way out of self-pity. Once I had a jewelry-brace, I had a new edgy visibility.

I am barely reconciled to the fact that I move quickly but write books slowly, even without the deaths of both a memory stick and a hard-drive that nearly terminated this project mid-point. *Surface Tensions* began as a manageable task. But it became unwieldy, its amplitude reflecting the conjunction of my own and others' thinking and writing about the body, and the proliferation of experiments, clinical advances and commercialization of the body and its parts. While I recovered from the loss of drafts and redrafts and retrieved my will, moved forward, collected more data, conducted more interviews and read ever more widely, my ideas mellowed, I like to think, and the book brewed. Each popular speculation about the boundaries of science – and debates about the ethics of the absence of such boundaries – added to the context in which all of us routinely accommodate our bodies and their limits. In 2011, the interventions to cure disease and reverse bodily dysfunction, and the ways that the biological body can be manipulated to change the course of individual lives, are now shaped by increasing optimism of potential discoveries in science and technology, rapid proven developments in interventions, and their expanded global commercialization.

Other kinds of restructuring and annotations of the body – tattoos, piercing, body building, cosmetic surgery – are now commonplace, not only in highly industrialized societies but globally. In September 1998 in Lyons, a team of French and Australian surgeons undertook the first transplant of a hand and forearm onto a New Zealand man whose own hand had been amputated fourteen years earlier. Sixteen months later, the same team conducted the first double hand transplant on a Frenchman who had lost his hands and forearms four years earlier, and in the spirit of the times, photographs of the transplant surgery were posted on the worldwide web. Three years later, this recipient was reported to be able to shave, use a fork and punch the buttons on his cell phone. By early 2006 the first full face transplant had eventuated, again in France; the second, two months later, took place in China. Worldwide, such medical news is sensationalized and the ethics of the practices and the outcomes for individuals are open to scrutiny. The original face transplant was framed by the problematics of heroic surgery – the woman had lost her face having been mauled by a dog, while she was comatose following an unsuccessful suicide attempt. But three years later, such transplantations have been repeated successfully, for those with access to high level care whose faces have been destroyed by gunshot or acid. These are the minority, of course. The more usual and often well publicized procedures are not face transplants, but serial cosmetic surgery on people seduced by the transformative promises of a surface change. Regular photo-essays in the popular press illustrate botched and excessive cosmetic surgery on celebrities.

Technological advances have shifted perceptions of disability and impairment only to some degree. As an example, consider the perverse debates about the alleged unfair advantage that Oscar Pistorius of South Africa might have, over able-bodied Olympic runners, because of his carbon-fiber prosthetic lower limbs. Yet in general, the mass media pays little attention to people who by birth, accident or illness must work with various bodily limitations and impairments, rarely questions the barriers to access and opportunity that are pervasive in all societies, and questions even less the general reluctance of inclusion and the priorities of modern medicine.

Significantly, in the early twenty-first century, globalization has accelerated people's familiarity with surgical and medical procedures and built up the research, technical capacity and health services in middle income countries. The body has become, far more so than earlier, a modest template for cultural and personal inscriptions. In Yueyang, a regional center in the impoverished province of Hunan, People's Republic of China, young people parade in the city center with tattoos, nose and eyebrow rings, and bright blue Mohawks, constructing and presenting identities of global youth that link them to their age mates in Singapore, London and Sydney while setting them sharply apart from their parents whose youth was shaped by the austerity of Maoist rule. Also in China, young women submit to leg-lengthening surgery in the belief that being tall will enhance their chances of prestigious employment and desirable marriages, and pageants such as the Miss Ugly Contest, with plastic surgery as its prize, reinforce the idea that bodily conformity is the gateway to success and happiness. Globally, people swallow vitamins, imbibe tonics, straighten or curl their hair, whiten or darken their skin, take extended lunch breaks for laser surgery to remove varicose veins or for botox injections to smooth out lines, and are persistently reminded of the all-importance of appearance by reality televisions shows such as Extreme Makeover. In Melbourne, Australia, with even less subtlety, body embellishments and procedures are undertaken live on radio and television: in real time, a woman has her nipples pierced and a young man has a 'Prince Albert' pierce (into and along his urethra). And, consistent with globalization, people travel for body modification at a discount. China's experience in leg-lengthening is now marketed internationally on the internet: on www.leg-lengthening. com, for example, the Beijing Institute of External Skeletal Fixation Technology claims innovative surgical advances in leg lengthening surgery that promise height increase with minimal risk and suffering. People can book on the internet and travel to India, Thailand, Malaysia, South Africa, Greece and Mexico, among other centers, not only for transsexual surgery – arguably the starting point of medical tourism – but for open heart surgery and more mundane procedures: hernia repair, gall bladder removal, hip and knee replacement, cataract removal and hysterectomy. Such surgical and medical holidays are routinely advertised as "first world treatment at third world prices" (Whittaker, Manderson, Cartwright 2010).

These developments provide a cultural backdrop to the necessary surgeries that shape this volume, surgeries that are undertaken for medical reasons and so are graver, less fanciful, but no less confrontational and transformative. *Surface Tensions* situates and tests theories of embodiment and wellbeing against empirical data from interviews with men and women who had had major surgery as a result of severe injury or disease. I commence with the premise that specific illnesses are identified, interpreted, and managed according to particular knowledge and belief systems, material circumstances, social institutions and social relations; these vary temporally and geographically. Illness and wellbeing are defined contextually. Bodily states, notions of the self, and relations of self to body are socially produced, and experiences and understandings of the body vary according to cultural context, social interactions and social forces. The body and mind, the corporeal self and the elusive mental being harbored within, are defined and understood by the ideas, structures and institutions of culture, race and ethnicity, religion, class, age and gender.

Acknowledgments

I like connections of time, place and people that allow for good fortune
and a sense of 'meant-to-be.' Behind this book are all kinds of synchron-
icities and happenstance. My hand is no longer encased in the grubby
scaffolding of an orthotic from a rehabilitation clinic, but supported by
a high-tech bracelet of aluminum, steel and leather, a synthetic work of
elegance, edge and provenance. It was made by Jason Patterson, one of
Stelarc's early collaborators: I thank Stelarc for the introduction, and
Jason for his artistry and continued willingness to repair and improvise.
The brace, developed from a combination of the principles of hand therapy
and anatomy, performance art and jewelry, gestures to films of robotics
and cyborgs, appropriately enough, given my references to films of this
genre throughout the book.

The preliminary work for this book commenced when I was a visit-
ing scholar in the Department of Anthropology, New School for Social
Research (now New School University), New York, 1997–1998; there,
I was fortunate to have Rayna Rapp as a colleague. In Bellagio, Italy, I
worked on a preliminary draft of this volume as a Scholar in Residence
at Villa Serbelloni, The Rockefeller Foundation and Conference Center.
I am indebted to the Rockefeller Foundation for the privilege of this stay
in an environment of exquisite beauty and incomparable intellectuality,
and to Gianna Celli and my fellow resident scholars and artists for their
warmth and conviviality. There, I met Wendy Woodson, leading to our
collaboration in the creation of the film, *Nerve* (2007). Our continuing
friendship inspires and challenges me to think in alternative ways about
representation, dissemination and translation. In Bellagio, too, I found a
clothing catalogue: the models in bandages and braces, their heads, tor-
sos and limbs trussed and pinned with improbable steel supports, midway
between my hand brace and scissorhands. With globalization, cyborg
imagery travels easily from the clinic to popular culture.

In Australia, between and after these sojourns offshore, I conducted research that has shaped this book with the generous support of the
Australian Research Council (ARC) through two small grants and, from
May 2002, through an ARC Federation Fellowship. My ideas on bodily
change and chronic conditions were tested in other research projects
funded by the ARC and by the National Health and Medical Research
Council, Australia, as they still are, and I acknowledge and am grateful for
the continued support of both these agencies. I commenced the empirical

research in 1998 while I was at The University of Queensland; I continued it after I moved to The University of Melbourne in1999, and finalized it at Monash University, where I moved in 2006.

Like all authors, behind me are numerous other people, some over decades, others more recently as the book gained form, who have been generous in time and spirit, often in elusive ways. To include some is to exclude others. Yet I do wish to acknowledge and formally thank a few of them. Geoffrey Ainsworth Harrison, Burton Singer, Richard Larkins and Ed Byrne had nothing to do with this book directly, but they have been truly generous in their support of me. Many of my doctoral students and colleagues contributed to this volume in some way; all provided me with regular opportunities to test out ideas and play with theories of the body in light of their own work as well as mine. Because they worked in related areas, Sarah Drew, Alex Gartrell, Keely Macarow and Susan Peake merit my especial thanks. Rae Smith, Liz Hoban, Susan Peake, Mollie Lane Jackson, Nittita Prasopa-Plasier and Kerry Hollier at different times introduced me to study participants, identified relevant literature, conducted interviews and managed the data. Narelle Warren routinely and with great generosity identified new scholarly articles, films and novels, and read and commented on the manuscript in time she didn't have. Anne Edmonds, Kathleen Nolan and Bharati Kalle brought calm and administrative order to my working life, creating for me the space I needed to write.

I am very grateful to Ju Gosling, Sharon Jones, Lucy Orta, Julie Rrap, Ariela Shavid and Stelarc for allowing me to publish their inspirational work. I am indebted to David Ades for his permission to include Melissa Jane Ades's work, to Sue Smith for reconstructing a digital copy of "One in Eleven" for its inclusion, to Brad Wilkinson, Alan Saunder, Teresa Gaudio and Sarah Walker, and to the librarians and curators responsible for various medical library and technology collections, all for their willing assistance. I thank Brad Nunn, Susan Cohn, Stelarc, Stephen Barker and Nancy Cato for their time, compelling stories and reflections. Judy Hogan and Noel Dillon of the Queensland Stoma Association were wonderfully open and enthusiastic about this work, and provided me with valuable introductions. I am indebted to the many other people who belonged to different consumer and health provider groups, who invited me to speak at their meetings about my research and shared their experiences and insights. And to all who shared with me your stories of suffering and triumph, and the prosaic and profound insights woven through them, my gratitude and admiration is immeasurable.

With great serendipity, this volume took a particular turn when I met Jennifer Collier of Left Coast Press Inc. I am indebted to her, and to Michael Jennings and Hannah Jennings, for their professionalism, talent, warmth and enthusiasm.

My brothers Richard, Roland and Desmond Manderson have provoked me for many years to think widely and creatively about corporeality, as through politics, sculpture, drama and the written text, and in everyday discourse, they, too, have pursued ideas about transubstantiation, transfiguration and transformation. My mother, Mardi Manderson, and my aunt, Beryl Hogarth, unwittingly provided me with tangible examples of bodily vulnerability and change.

And always: Pat, Tobi and Kerith nurture my soul and give me great joy.

Lenore Manderson
Melbourne, June 2011

Prologue 🙼

Perdita's Story

Perdita and I met through a work colleague. She was an active member of a support group for men and women who had an ostomy. This is the creation of an opening, most commonly to divert and expel waste when the bladder, urethra, anus, or rectum is unable to function, although for some, such as those with throat cancer, a tracheostomy enables them to breath. Stomas are a life-saving, necessary change. My colleague thought I would find in Perdita a receptive and interested participant. She was loquacious, energetic, frank and funny; we formed a warm friendship. She brought me to local meetings, introduced me to others who had had a stoma, invited me to seminars and conferences, solicited articles. At the same time we talked, with lots of incidental chats, and ten hours on a tape as she built up her own complicated story, managing the narrative process as well as content.

Perdita was a taxation accountant working with a small group of business clients. Her marriage was languid but familiar; her children secure; her friends trusty and supportive. She was 49 and in relatively good health – she swam, she played golf, she ate well – when she went to see her gynecologist prior to a curette, and mentioned that she thought she had a hemorrhoid, and asked him to check her out because it was uncomfortable, she was constipated, and had some bleeding. He agreed he'd cauterize the hemorrhoid at the same time as the curette. When she woke up from the anesthetic after the curette, her gynecologist was sitting on the bed beside her, and told her that he thought she had cancer in the rectum. The multiple indignities began.

The preparation for the colonoscopy involved a full day fast, taking in specific liquids only, then from early evening the bowel lavage, a powder mixed into four liters of water, defined by its manufacturers as having a "mild salty taste" and by Perdita, among others, as tasting "disgusting." The mixture is drunk steadily, a full glass every ten minutes, precipitating continual explosive diarrhea until the colon is clean, the stools clear, and the body ready for exploration. The next day Perdita presented to the hospital. She was given an analgesic and sedated, and the colonoscope was inserted up her anus, through the larger colon, and into the small intestine. But the colon was not clean enough, and so the view impaired. A week later Perdita repeated the lavage preparation and the colonoscopy. This time, a few polyps were removed and biopsies were taken of other uncertain lesions. The pathology was positive, and a week later, Perdita was booked for surgery. Perdita entered the hospital knowing she would require a major resection of her large colon, but she lost most of her bowel. She awoke with a permanent colostomy. And so she began to come to terms with the permanence of the stoma, the odor and texture of the waste, care of the opening and prevention of lesions; she learned to monitor the bag, to empty it regularly, to avoid leakages and burst bags, and to modify her diet to control odor, gas and noise:

> The stoma is very fragile and you have to treat it carefully, like when you've got to wipe it say ten to fifteen times a day, you know, that can aggravate the skin, can aggravate the stoma if you are filling the bag and, well, it can start it bleeding, and so I have to wipe very gently. But it is just those tiny little blood cells and you are just bursting a little blood vessel and it is not, you know, all that dangerous but if you are very, very rough you can end up with all sorts of problems … I mean, you can scratch yourself, and get fecal material into a cut or a raw bit of skin so you end up infecting yourself… you have to pack the area with a particular paste, get the appliance on, have it stay there to collect the material as it expels. Infections are pretty rife with ostomates, I would say.

Meanwhile, Perdita's personal relationships began to unravel. Her children, who had thought her "infallible," were frightened by her cancer and its explicit threat to her life, embarrassed by the ostomy and the bag: "they didn't want to know about it." Her relationship with her husband shifted quickly, too, from indifference and apathy, to revulsion and withdrawal from his standpoint, and to anger and hurt from hers. So she faced radiotherapy almost alone, as those she trusted most withdrew. Perdita had radiotherapy for five days a week for five weeks – and while she felt that she had no real problems with her skin, experienced neither nauseous nor diarrhea, she felt degraded:

I was just so frightened. Radiotherapy frightened me. I think it's the unknown. I mean, your dignity just goes out the door. There was a chair as you walked in the door, and you took everything off there and there was supposed to be a sheet on that chair and you had to walk from that chair to that machine. And they're all standing around looking at you. I've got to lie on a table, my backside up in the air and the doctors drawing all over my backside with a texta pen. And that's got to stay there for the whole time you have your treatment. You're not allowed to wash that area or anything. You know, all these things you have to find out. Me, someone who was so fussy about showering every day – makeup, clothes, everything – and then all of a sudden, here I was with young people (medical staff) around me, with my backside up in the air. It was just so degrading. Your dignity, you can just forget that. Having a baby is supposed to be – you're supposed to be blooming – it's supposed to be the greatest ecstasy of your life, you know. Having surgery when you're sick is different. It didn't even worry me though, I think because, first of all, I was operated on so quickly, and then the radiotherapy was so soon after that. I didn't even have time to come to terms with an appliance on my stomach and my image and the way I felt.

By the time the radiotherapy was over, Perdita had left her job and found a new one with a smaller company; she had left her family home, separated from her husband, and settled into a new apartment. A year later, she was divorced. And she learned to work around the boundaries of her body and to quickly acquire an etiquette of body management to avoid the worst bodily and social effects of having a stoma:

> All of us carry our appliances or we should, anyway, our wipes so that we get to wipe around the area, carry a disposable bag to put in the bin and our own tissues and that sort of thing to avoid infection. Because infection in the stoma is horrific. And antibiotics can give us diarrhea, they can also constipate us, and if you have a stoma and constipation, you're in excruciating pain. And if we get constipation and a blockage, it could mean a trip to the hospital for a start if you can't get rid of the blockage yourself through massage or things like that … and when you go to hospital and they put you on a drip if that doesn't clear it then it is surgery … I'm lucky, I've got most of my bowel because the cancer was down very, very low in the colon, while some colostomates

might have lost three or four feet of their bowel, but you have to be careful. Some colostomates irrigate, but it depends where the stoma is placed. Irrigating takes about forty-five minutes and then you can go for forty-eight hours with just a little plug, just a little tiny patch, and you don't have this bag of feces around. But I cant, according to my doctor, because I have what they call a transcending stoma. You just have to put up with it.

Perdita continued on this theme of self-knowledge, body management and surveillance at another interview:

You have to put up with it. There could be ten of us sitting in this room talking to you now, and they will all say, yes I can eat anything, that's fine, they can even drink anything. But the side effect is that they have a full bag all the time, they are full of gas, they have odor, and if they want to live with that, that's their business. But for the life of me, I mean, there are so many foods – as I have said to you before in the last interview – so many foods we eat that do not digest well, things like peanuts to watch because they can cause blockage, peas – the skin of the pea doesn't digest. I would not want to run the risk of creating an obstruction; I can do without peas. If I can avoid problems by not eating certain things, I will. I am exactly the same as everyone else except I do have a stoma. I still feel self-conscious, though, especially if I get a bit of diarrhea and the bag started to fill up rather rapidly, it is like a balloon going up. Once the air starts to get into it, it expands … some days I get really angry and other days I think I feel like the hunchback of Notre Dame gone wrong, you know. Anger, yes, anger comes into it, for most of us I think.

Then, resuming golf and trying to establish a life outside of stoma surgery and cancer, Perdita met Erik. She avoided telling him that she had a stoma until they were about to become intimate, and by that time, despite her secrecy about her health, they had established a relationship of trust, and Perdita felt comfortable enough to explain, although still – always – to hide the stoma and the bag. They were fortunate, too; their ideas of the etiquette of bodily communication and the specifics of love-making converged:

I am a touching person and he and I, we'd be in the middle of the street, and cuddle and things like that. And a couple of times I'd break off because I thought, oh, he can feel it. And he knew what I was doing and he said to me, don't do that, because, he said, it doesn't matter.

You are you, this does not take any shape or form, it's there, it's part of you – that's it, I'm happy to cuddle all of you. And then I never worried about it again. I knew that there would be somebody out there, one day, who would want me and I would deal with the colostomy when it happened. I didn't worry about it. I couldn't afford to anyway, because stress is your worst enemy when you've had cancer. But I hadn't slept with another man for years, so that was another thing, because as you would be aware, inside you start to get smaller and smaller and tighter and tighter, so when we first made love it was quite uncomfortable. And while he's very passionate in his lovemaking, he's not one to let his mouth wander all over you. All around the breast area, yes, but anywhere else, no. That's a no-no. So the way we started off, I mean, I knew it was never going to be a problem because of the way he preferred to make love. That suited me down to the ground. I mean I – it didn't worry me that he wasn't doing these extra things.

But as she told me of this love story, Perdita was still managing both the narrative process and content:

I was every day learning something different about colostomy. But it didn't worry me – I thought, I'm alive, I mean I can't ask for any more, but for what I was going through, now I'd be dead. But the thing that I'm just about to tell you now is that in January last year, I had breast cancer. I've also had a mastectomy. My right breast is a prosthesis. So do you understand now how special my partner is, and how special, I guess, I am? I know that I'm a really good subject for this project for what you're doing. I think it's just brilliant. And when I spoke to you, I thought, I've got to talk to this lady because I'm sure I can help.

As described earlier, Perdita reflects on her husband's 'specialness' because she has had both a colostomy and a mastectomy, both of which are confronting to the person affected and to others around them, and she reflects on her role as a research participant. For Perdita, the hardest point in managing breast cancer was chemotherapy and its side effects:

One of the physical sides of chemotherapy is hair loss, of course; the other is, you become very sick, um, you know you lose your appetite also, and it gives us [ostomates] diarrhea. So you have got what I term as chronic diarrhea, through the chemotherapy, because you have no control over it, you can't. There is nothing to take to avoid that, it is just one of the side effects. You know, for three months, like for instance if I would have had to have it, I would have had to have the dosage for

three months, I would have just been so sick, and I remember the day
I was operated on, and I remember the day the doctor said you can go
home tomorrow, but you are going to have to have treatment. The day
I was operated on, I was the most positive thinker and I was fine, and
I will get through this, life goes on…

And so, while Perdita managed the aftermath now of breast cancer as
well as bowel cancer, a breast prosthesis as well as a stoma, she and Erik
found ways to maintain their intimacy without embarrassment. Despite
her tactile openness, Perdita insists that the light is off when they make
love. While she acknowledged that "kissing the body is one way of expressing love and sexuality also includes kissing," she always covers her right
side, her right chest with its mastectomy scar as well as her stoma and bag.
And despite her optimism and irreverence, she faces difficulties with and
as a result of her body every day:

> I am as happy as a pig in mud now. I have Erik, and although these last
> three years have been a bit heavy at times, I don't think I get near as
> angry. But sometimes … like the other day, I just burst into tears. The
> loss of control is clearly one of the hardest things because it strips you of
> your adulthood… the awfulness of being our age and just losing control.

Erik grounds her. He keeps an eye out for her, and keeps her positive.
Sometimes, Perdita says, she feels everyone around her can smell her, and
is staring at her. But even at times of acute embarrassment – with leakage
or a burst bag, for example – he reassures her, "it's all right, it's all right,
don't get upset, it's all right." He knows how she feels, Perdita explains.
But even Erik cannot address her recurrent questions of risk, cause and
responsibility. These are questions she asked her doctor and the nurses
the morning after the surgery for colorectal cancer, ones she returned to
after her mastectomy, ones that recur in moments of awkwardness and at
times of reflection:

> I started to get quite angry. I mean, I started throwing questions
> left, right and center: Why did this happen to me? I have done this,
> this, this, and this through my life, you know, and as far as I can see I
> have done everything right. So why has it happened to me? I thought
> I was continually doing the right thing. I was never an aggressive
> person or anything. I just couldn't understand it. What have I done
> in my life to deserve this? I really don't lay the blame on anyone or
> anything, but that's probably because the last three years have been
> so good for me…

1

The Body as Subject

Our life shatters, our plans collapse, and beyond us as individuals, the various social organizations appear rigid, closed, hostile – they would have to be blown apart. In us, or around us, the onset of disability creates a disorganization that is both concrete and social. But from this vantage point we perceive yet another disorganization, much deeper and more painful, the disorganization of our acquired understandings, of our established values. (Stiker 1999:3)

I kept projecting life into the future. But with the uncertainty of how long I've got, it didn't matter anymore; there was no future. It has been very liberating to make the most of it. Like, if I'm not happy with my life, I've got the power to do something about it today, to make whatever I have got great. Yet control is an illusion. And even when I slip back into trying to control things and have them the way they should be to keep life manageable, there is no control. I'm paralyzed over everything. (Janice, research participant)

This book is about catastrophes of the body. It is not about immediate crises, but about life afterwards; not about unfolding dramas of serious medical conditions, the urgent surgery to excise an aggressive cancer or to save a limb crushed by a fallen bar of steel, but rather, about how people see themselves when they cease to be at the center of such dramas. When the urgency to maintain life has passed, when the role of inpatient is over, when rehabilitation is complete, how do people come simply to live with their new changed bodies? How do they make sense of embodied change, recreate their lives to accommodate new constraints and contingencies, rebuild the self in a new casing? If the body is "a coat to the soul" – as one of my research participants, Janice, suggested to me – is the soul, or the self, unscathed when the fabric is frayed and the seams re-stitched?

Personal identity is constituted in various, complicated ways, including by inherited, ascribed and acquired qualities and characteristics – age, race, sexuality, gender and marital status, for example – and the cultural meanings attached to these. The physical body, its capacity and functions, contribute to this identity. Drew Leder (1990) argues that by separating the body and mind, people are able to maintain their sense of core identity and personhood, so that this identity is contingent neither on body function nor appearance, nor vulnerable to bodily changes. But not everyone holds to these ideas of the separation of body and mind. If the body and mind are somehow consubstantial or enlaced, then questions emerge on the impact of change to one domain on the other. How is the self reconstructed when people experience profound negative corporeal change? What does it mean to be a person living in or with a body with indelibly changed functions, if the body and mind defy segregation? How do people conceive of their own personhood or maintain an idea of an essential self that is either salient to changes in or, alternatively, independent of body form, structure and function?

People face practical, ideational and perceptual challenges as they seek to make sense of necessary yet often undesirable embodied changes. They struggle with the ambivalence inherent in this task as they reconcile with and adapt to physical differences and changes in function that derive from illness, injury or surgery, and as they relate these to their sense of self. They negotiate, or battle with, the inconsistencies between body and mind that play out at individual and societal levels.

Descartes's fingerprints are ubiquitous in any discussion of body and mind, as in the sustained scholarly interest in body and self. For the ideas that derive from his distinction between body and mind have been remarkably enduring, despite objections even from his contemporary Spinoza and subsequently about the relative fixity or fluidity of this relationship, and of the particularity and the cultural variability of ideas of body/mind and body/spirit (MacCormack 1982; Csordas 1994). In attempting to explain the appeal of ideas of the divide between the two, Drew Leder (1990) proposes the idea of bodily absence, the usual lack of awareness by people of their bodies, bodily parts, and the execution of functions. "Human experience," he begins his book, "is incarnated. I receive the surrounding world through my eyes, my ears, my hands. The structure of my perceptual organs shapes that which I apprehend. And it is via bodily means that I am capable of responding" (1). Leder sees the presence of the body as paradoxical and conceptually elusive, since one's own body is "rarely the thematic object of experience" (1). We don't feel our eyes seeing, or feel our ears hearing. Instead, we interpret our capacity to see because of images before us. We identify the pathological through variations to the individual norm. There is no objectivity, for not all of us see the same thing (e.g., through variations in stereoscopic vision, astigmatism, color blindness and so on). Similarly, what we hear proves we do hear, and the pathological is a consequence of signs that counter our own assumptions, because others claim to hear what we cannot, or we hear what others cannot: ringing tones or voices, for instance, or physical or mental disturbances.

Eco (2000:56) takes a similar standpoint:

> We are the ones who think that our leg (in articulating at the knee) can describe some angles, from 180 to 45 degrees, but it *cannot* describe an angle of 360 degrees. The leg – for what little a leg can be said to "know" – is unaware of any limits and is aware only of possibilities.

Eco is writing metaphorically. He is concerned neither with the reality of a leg that can or cannot articulate, nor with any other body part limited by its original structure or subsequent constraints. His concern, rather, is with limits to being, and the limits to our imagination of possible modes of being – "the limit is in our desire, in our reaching out for absolute freedom" (56). Yet in pursuing the idea of potential and resistance, he captures neatly how we are constrained by prejudices of the relationship of body to mind, and the extrapolations that we therefore make from physical appearance and function to capacity and capability. Changes to the body – the inability to flex a leg at all, for instance, or the lack of a leg – create existential, social and practical dilemmas for the person so affected, and for others with whom she or he interacts. But at the same time, the body is limited in its self-perception. The workings of internal organs are rarely felt. One cannot see the small of one's back.

In pursuing ideas of bodily irregularity, anomaly and identity, I have found it helpful in writing this book to revisit and draw on the work particularly of Drew Leder, on the earlier work of biological philosopher Georges Canguilhem (1991 [1943]) and on the more recent writing of historian Henri-Jacques Stiker (2001). The writings of other more familiar anthropologists and sociologists gird these ideas. Goffman (1959, 1963), Douglas (1966, 1973) and Foucault (1973, 1978), for example, provide particular insight into the sociology and social history of the body. These works emerged mainly in the 1960s and 1970s, concurrently with a scholarly literature and political projects on corporeality, identity and the construction of self, on race and ethnicity, gender and sexuality, and disability. They were succeeded by a wide range of publications on bodies, multiply conceptualized and diversely theorized, and on the reproduction, construction and exigencies of physical bodies. The foundational work of these early authors is central to analyzing bodily transformation, decline and reinvention.

Leder's project in *The Absent Body* was to explain the endurance of the distinction between body and mind. He argues that the body is taken for granted when it is healthy; it becomes a presence in the mind only when there is discernible visible or felt pathology. A body in pain, a febrile and sweating body, a fetid wound, is present; without pain or fever, corporeal awareness recedes. Yet this awareness is fragmentary, Leder argues, for sensitivity of the body as present is heightened with dysfunction because of the "very absence of a desired or ordinary state, and as a force that stands opposed to the self" (1990:4). The body in its entirety is taken for granted, even with bodily dysfunction; as one part of the body gains salience, the rest of the body slips into disregard. Healthiness and normality are states in which one notices the body as little as possible (Canguilhem 1991).

But at the same time, I suggest, presence and absence, and the pathologies that influence these shifting states of awareness, can be immeasurably close. Bodily dysfunction need not indicate disease, and disease need not be observed. Viral infection, parasite infestation, or the growth of a cancer in the body, for instance, rarely manifests early; rather, it is the consequences of disease or infection on the organs or viscera that are felt, often when pathology is well-established. One does not *feel* cancer; rather, the abnormalities of cells are objectively observed through palpation, ultrasound, MRI (magnetic resonance imaging), X-ray or laboratory test. But parts of the interior body are routinely observed and felt, not because of pain, but though ingestion, inhalation, reflux, studied concentration or deeply meditative breathing. Conversely, the absence of corporeal, sensory or perceptual dysfunction is not evidence of positive functioning; hence the wariness of individuals in remission from cancer, its possible return is an ever-present fear. And, in contrast, the presence of an absence is precisely that: deafness is a state of difference that is not felt (as deafness). Disability politics negotiates this very territory of embodied difference and capacity. Symptoms and dysfunction may suggest underlying pathology, but these are not equivalent.

These generalizations inevitably overstate the commonality of experiences of the body. Cultural, personal, age and gender differences, at least, inform our self-consciousness about embodiment and bodily functions. Leder may be right that the body is absent for men in good health for much of their adult life, although this ignores the invasive embodied responses of the sexual body. And women, for a major portion of their adult life, routinely experience their bodies as cyclically present. We tacitly observe our bodies and functions, flows, floods, aches, heaviness, twinges and fullness, proving normality as an ordinary *present* body. Yet at the same time, individual women challenge the universality of norms on the basis of appearance, comportment and performance; at various points they feel the twinge of ovulation, the fullness of breasts, the heaviness of their belly, or the commencement of the flow of menstrual blood into their vagina. Such bodily sensations are felt independently of any discomfort; they indicate a normal body. In contrast, the absence of or variation in such signs highlights a 'normal' anomaly – menopause or pregnancy – but also dysfunction or disorder, flagging unexpected anovulation, for instance.

In other cases, manifestations of the physical body may be perceived as neither positive nor negative. Sweating, sneezing, itchiness, changes in breathing and pulse, changes in sensation or gait may vary in their ephemerality, persistence, and the degree to which we are mindful of and interpret them, but their presence is not necessarily pathological, and they may precipitate neither self-conscious monitoring nor reflection. Our awareness of our bodies is usually muted. But the body is ever present. A person without self-consciousness interacts with his or her body through habitual as much as autonomic action: blinking purposively, rubbing an eye to clear it, shifting our weight, clearing our throat, scratching and so on, without conscious premeditation and without the need to see what we are doing. We recognise peristaltic pressure and act upon it. We are always doing to or interacting with our bodies: sometimes intentionally (nose blowing, hair brushing, cleaning teeth), sometimes mindlessly (scratching, pinching, sucking teeth, licking lips, chewing nails, and so on). In moving, interacting with and tending to our bodies in various ways, we arouse bodily perceptions (the firmness of a shirt or shoes, the sensitivity of skin from a smooth shave), and we react to corporeal intrusions, such as the sound and feel of a burp, a swallow or a cough, or the awareness of dampness from sweat, vaginal discharge or urine. None of these conditions needs cause pain nor indicate disease; many have nothing to do with volition; few are necessarily unpleasant. We take our bodies for granted, attending to them only when there is unpredictable marked discomfort, pain, anomaly or distress. We are, therefore, far more attuned to and used to working with our body than Leder, Canguilhem, and others writing in this vein allow. We rely on perceptive, kinesthetic and proprioceptive responses to act in ways that allow us to respond to our environment and to sustain an awareness of bodily boundaries (Leder 1990:176–177, fn 27) without self-consciousness (178, fn 62). Bourdieu's idea of habitus and Casey's of "body memories of habits" are useful here. We experience our bodies and so embody ways of experiencing the world. While dysfunction or dys-appearance can lead to hyperawareness – pain can be overwhelming – changes in affectivity, motility or proprioception rapidly become a normal part of the normal body. At the same time, we adapt to and absorb tools that fuse with the body. Glasses are an example, but somewhat passive; the use of instruments that require more active incorporation is a better example, where the person has to adapt to the equipment.

Ordinary leisurely and productive body regimes require people to engage with their bodies to learn new functions or activities – to write, type, swim, ride a bike, or play a musical instrument; in time many of the actions involved in these processes become intuitive – this is habitus (Bourdieu 1977). Body disciplines such as yoga, Pilates and Feldenkrais, in contrast, demand self-consciousness of the body, so that the practitioner concentrates on isolating body parts such as muscles and functions such as breathing that are usually autonomic, taken-for-granted, or undifferentiated. Teasing out the sequences of thought and action to achieve a particular effect, or to differentiate cause, effect and directionality, can be tortuous, since even the simplest cognitive and physical actions are imbricated. Yet not all people have the pre-existing functions or capacity to undertake these tasks. They may have limited or no vision, they may lack the flexibility to bend or stoop, or lack a thumb to grasp. Through disease or injury, they may not have full executive function. They may lack the cognitive capacity or linguistic competence to name an object. They may have never had some of these functions, or they may have lost function, near instantaneously or gradually.

Technologies of the body, like physical states, can be imperceptible, mutable and fluid. A dental implant, an inter-uterine device, a hip replacement or a stent may be largely or entirely unfelt. Other instruments, tools and prosthetics, such as a pacemaker, glasses, a brace or a hearing aid, may be incorporated into the body schema even if visible and/or removable. A person learns to adapt to equipment, allowing the body to merge with foreign technologies. For instance, a person fitted with a prosthetic arm following an amputation must learn to use his or her shoulder and back

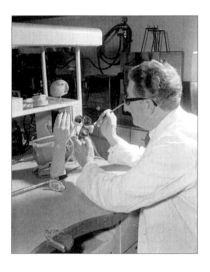

Figure 1.1 Technician preparing a facial prosthesis; 1971. Photograph by Laurie Richards. Courtesy of Museum Victoria.

muscles in order to 'work' the prosthesis, and doing so, he or she comes to integrate these movements and the actions of the prosthesis into his or her body schema and habitus. But while such technologies are incorporated, the simplest unproblematically, they tamper with identity and sense of self. So, too, do specific histories of the body and mind. Life threatening illnesses, sexual experience and expression, reproduction and parenting, and the acuity or flatness of sensory perceptions, all in distinct ways shape individual self-representation. Family and other social relationships, and various historical, social and economic factors, likewise bring different meanings to the body. In contrast to Leder's examples, therefore, the absence of familiar bodily signs, rather than the presence of atypical signs, flags pathology.

Unless we have a specific bodily or health condition from birth or infancy that early forces a detour in expectations of our body and life course, parents and others assume that we will be healthy and able-bodied for most or all of our lives; we internalize this supposition. When this is not the case, the effects can be profoundly disruptive. Those affected must adjust to their changed flesh and skills, change how they manage bodily functions and actions, revise the rhythms and content of everyday activities, reorganize domestic and negotiate public space, redefine personal relationships, rethink life directions. Physical changes place new finiteness on bodies, and, as suggested above, people must redefine who they are to themselves and to others. People who have had major surgery or an accident remain to a degree 'sick' in the public imagination, either because the appurtenances of rehabilitation and function (e.g. wheelchairs, prosthetic limbs) are visible or because of the profound stigma when the cause of debility is made public. The body is a metaphor of the social world (Sontag 1978), but the social world, its structures and institutions, leaves physical imprints on the body, mnemonics of global and local moral, social and political relationships. People must, in whatever ways make sense for them, accommodate bodily exigencies, establish their own capabilities, and rewrite their futures. These social aftershocks following bodily changes impact on and interact with other defining components of personhood.

Sudden disruptions to the physical body create different problems in autobiography than those that emerge in the case of gender, sexuality, ethnicity or other aspects of identity. The narrative frameworks for sexual identity, for example, do not work when the biographic turn is dramatic. While the known etiology of disease provides some people with retrospective logic, particularly when they embrace the self-blame of neo-liberal philosophy (*I smoked, I didn't eat the right foods*), there is no precedence in the everyday experience of contemporary industrialized societies that allows an individual to anticipate catastrophe, nor is there a template by which to reconstruct and recast a personal story along the lines of *this is my true self*. As Arthur Frank (1990) suggested in his reflections on cancer, a person faced with sudden bodily change instead draws on narratives of restitution and quest; unable to control the willful (i.e. diseased) body, he or she seeks to re-establish what is understood to be the former relationship with the body, and to find a new, positive way of accounting, existentially, for an otherwise unwelcome turn. As I illustrate in this book, the possibility of restitution is limited for a person whose corporeality is transformed through surgery; he or she must resolve the inconsistencies between wanting to recover his or her body and/or control it and being unable to do so. Gaining and claiming new personal qualities is one adaptive strategy that offers some reconciliation to embodied change.

Any bodily change ushers an existential reckoning. People whose bodies change in undesired and unpredictable ways must rethink themselves, challenging conventional ideas of the integrity of the body and mind in order to understand their selves in light of physical reconfiguration and confinement. While increasingly people hold to the idea of the integration of body-mind, the popular persistence of ideas of dualism is a functional adaptation in the face of embodied limits. If "I" is the mind (or in or of the mind), and the body the site *merely* wherein I dwell, then the loss of a body part or function inhibits but does not erode the self; for this reason, as I illustrate, individuals are able to speak of being normal despite bodily change. As noted earlier, Leder makes this point in his phenomenological account of the appeal and pervasiveness of Cartesian dualism, in which a body that is ill or in pain becomes a "thematic object" or "alien presence" (79) in the way of ordinary activities, actions and relations to the extent that it presents itself "as a problem to be solved, whether on the plane of ordinary experience or philosophical reflection" (132). The standpoint of people with bodily disruptions, as I will illustrate, demonstrates this. People grapple with ideas of the essence of being, with tensions between corporeality and intellect, body and soul. They do so often in prosaic ways. Many would find philosophizing about the nature of being an indulgence, and are concerned simply to get on with the business of living. People who have experienced profound body change must conceptualize their bodies, reconstruct their sense of self, and rehabituate. They reinvent the use of their body and, in the process of adaptation, internalize and (in Leder's terms) make the present absent. The impediment is worked with, not against – is incorporated in the body schema at the level of neurology, and so in terms of everyday bodily actions and habitus. In arguing – as many do – that they are apart from the body and its boundaries, however, people insist upon personhood beyond the limits of the flesh.

The Cultural Backdrop

Science and cultures of the body consistently interact. The sustained emphasis in the first decade of the twenty-first century on body maintenance, renewal and embellishment builds on the constant rewards of scientific discovery, technical advance and fantastic possibility. Conversely, contemporary academic interest in the body and society, biology and corporeality reflects this popular interest, the increasing demand for access to technology, and the elective applications of medical products and knowledge. The dramatic growth in the use of new reproductive technologies to override biological timelines is one example; so is the cosmetic application of Botulism toxin (Botox) and collagen to create a temporary illusion that aging itself has been defeated, or the use of surgery to address psychological crises, vanity or fashion, or the optimistic deposits in umbilical cord blood and adult stem cell banks as a hedge against possible degenerative disease. Public debates about embryonic stem cell research, life support, xenotransplantation, and cloning feed into popular nineteenth and twentieth century discourses of the ethics of science, while illustrating the politics of the articulation of science and commerce. State and popular morality, not industry nor technical skill, has braked many of the developments in these areas.

Questions of bodily maintenance and change have long exercised scholars from various standpoints and disciplines, including from philosophy, anthropology, sociology and psychology, and natural science,

Figure 1.2 Left: Stelarc, *Involuntary Body/Third Hand*. Melbourne; 1990. Diagram by Stelarc. Right: Stelarc, *Handwriting*. Maki Gallery, Tokyo; 1982. Photograph by Keisuke Oki. Courtesy of Stelarc.

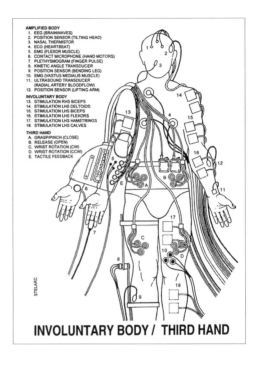

medical engineering and clinical practice. Paradigmatic and epistemological differences still distinguish biological and social accounts of the nature of the body and the relationships that exist between psychological state and corporeality. Contemporary social scientists understand the body to be both biological and social. How these properties or sets of properties interact and interrelate, each changing the character of the other, is a continuing question. Yet there is growing recognition of the complex interplay of mind and physical body, and the contribution of environmental factors and emotion to the development of disease – the links between economic status and social stress, smoking and low birth weight, for example, or between health and social capital, emotional status and physical health. Diseases that result in visible changes in physiology and biology, that are believed to cause changes in cognition or intellectual ability, or are communicable (leprosy, tuberculosis and HIV, for example), have always been subject to complex cultural constructs and interpretive frameworks. Many of these conditions are imbued with negative connotations that, through metaphor, social interaction and the institutionalization of stigma, constrain the social and economic participation of affected individuals and so

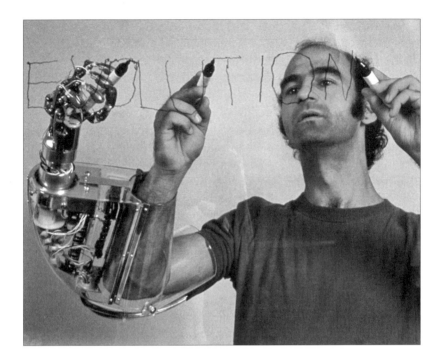

limit their life choices (Goffman 1963). So, too, social and psychological life can produce organic changes – hence the recent and rapid development of integrative research fields such as psychoneuroimmunology and psychoneuroendocrinology.

But we have an uneven knowledge of the etiology of disease, the development of interventions, and the lived experiences of people with such conditions. Social research on ill and well bodies is not new, of course; anthropologists have always been concerned with the body and body matter in relation to both the prosaic and metaphysical. Witchcraft and sorcery, religion and ritual, health and healing practice, birth and death are conventional considerations in ethnography, even when the focus is predetermined somewhat by the economics and politics of knowledge and the bodies (by age and gender) of both the researched and the researchers. Indeed, in exploring questions of corporeality and body maintenance, and the societal imperative to manage physical bodies, practices and desires, many early works, such as the classical studies of Rivers (1927), Evans-Pritchard (1937) and Malinowski (1922), anticipated the debates central to much contemporary scholarship.

Early theorizing about bodily practices drew attention to the structural importance rather than personal meanings of bodily governance, that is, on the relevance of body practices to the constitution of society (Leach 1967; Douglas 1973; Blacking 1977; Loudon 1977; Douglas 1978 [1966]). By the 1980s, social, cultural and medical anthropology had produced significant work on bodies, illness, healers and healing practices, resulting in a rich corpus of work that makes synthesis problematic. Anthropological interest in embodiment, inspired by European philosophers, notably Merleau-Ponty (1962; 1968:45), is most relevant to this work. As already noted, the body is a source of, and the vehicle for, understanding experience, including experience of the body itself. People reconstruct and refigure who they are, making sense of the relationship of self and body with shifts in personal circumstances. But as Foucault (1977, 1978) famously argued, individual bodies are governed and shaped by specific political, economic and social contexts, and the relationships of individuals in context.

Tattooing is one example of this. Tattooing is well understood as occurring in most societies not as adornment alone, but as public notation of an individual's affiliation, identity, social responsibility and/or for magical protection. This is true not only of customary tattoos in small scale societies. The tattoo on the arm of a survivor of a death-camp very particularly positions that person in time and place; so, too, do self-crafted tattoos on the knuckles of young Australians and Britons. Likewise, circumcision indelibly marks the body and the person in terms of allegiance, identity and status. Rules related to covering, controlling, and containing the body literally and symbolically shape everyday social relations. Cultural apparatus is applied to bodies as material items, marking them as social tools. Other bodily markings, varying in time and place, similarly reflect context, institutions and social relations: paralysis from polio, stunting, vision or hearing loss, the pits of small-pox or, indeed, the scars of inoculation are embodied testimonies of inequalities between countries and the unevenness of the incidence, prevention and control of infections at given moments in history. The suture line from carpal tunnel surgery on the wrist of a modern office worker and the scarred lungs of a miner are similarly embodiments of unequal relations of production.

These inequalities feed into cultural attitudes towards bodies and bodily diversity, and determine how people make sense of these corporeal reminders, perceive of and cater to bodily wants and needs, understand ailments, prevent and repair the body, and seek assistance. Cultural ideas about the body also influence how people interact on the basis of physical appearance. Health, illness and disability, normality and pathology are socially and culturally construed. Canguilhem (1991:22) uses Jasper's notion of health as the absence of illness, but he also acknowledges the importance of context in health and normality. Pathology is not an absolute, he argues; rather, it exists only in relation to a given, defined situation as 'well enough' – that is, not ill – and so both normal in a particular setting and normative in respect to this and other situations (196). Aging and frailty instantiate this, for regardless of bodily and mental function and capability, a person is 'normal' (and not living in a pathological state) to the extent that there is consistency in relation to other older people and to how they were before. Biological variety and change are inevitable; thus pathology can include the absence of change at organic and phenomenological levels. Consequently, while technical capability and access to goods and services influence outcomes, by determining normality, societal values largely create and reinforce hierarchies of ability and disability, as Davidson (2009) has most recently depicted. The conditions and surgical outcomes on which I focus in the volume – primarily amputation, stoma surgery, mastectomy and kidney transplants – provide rich territory to interrogate the cultural and social construction of the body. As those affected are acutely aware, to be considered healthy and productive – the two aligned in the social imagination – and accorded full social membership requires that people are in control of and can take care of their own physical bodies. But many conditions inhibit mobility, limit the ability to self-care, and may leave people insensate, physically dependent, with variable energy, and vulnerable. Those who have been ill, who have undergone life-saving surgery, or who live with a refractory body must deal with bodily exigency and limit, replacing old habitus with self-conscious management. This is hard enough. However, unruly embodiment is often interpreted not as an artifact of a physical event, but as the corporeal symbol of a fundamental failure or decay of character. Loss of physical mobility and autonomy is typically only the first step, for with physical impairment people lose public acknowledgement of their (continued) intellectual or mental agency. With this metamorphosis from being well to being disabled, the social body is often questioned; the mind may also be seen as out of control. Scars, pock marks, slurred speech, a curved spine or a limp is read by others not only as a summary history of an individual body but also as symbolic of the person as a whole, of his or her character and social standing, capacity and capability, sexuality, gender identity, and intrinsic worth as a human being. Stigma draws on this alignment of body and mind.

While the processes of stigma, discrimination and social exclusion lead others to infer social from physical incapacity, these beliefs are internalized; people so affected are mindful of how others see them and must reassess their own assumptions of the meanings of particular bodies. Social and personal accommodation to physical disability can be difficult both in resource-poor and relatively wealthy settings, but disability is exacerbated in the absence of the resources to improve infrastructure, provide services and ensure social safety nets. Personal, community and national poverty compounds the difficulties of adjustment to acquired embodied changes, stripping people of the possibilities of regaining ability, maximizing capability, and continuing to participate fully in society.

Cultural values also shape the salience of specific conditions. In various cultural settings, personal responsibility is implicated in many conditions affecting women, including fetal loss, sexually transmitted infections and certain cancers, and in some cases, men's afflictions, too, may be attributed to women's refractory behavior. In industrialized societies, anorexia illustrates the entangling of the social and physical body, self and society, through tensions concerning body image and diet, and although there are various etiologies, some women seek to control bodily desire (appetite) by controlling the behavior (eating), perversely losing control over their bodies as they seek to establish it. Those involved in this war against the self are caught irrevocably in the paradoxes of self-control (Warin 2003). Female urinary incontinence also illustrates dilemmas of the social and physical body (Mitteness and Barker 1995; Peake, Manderson, Potts 1999; Isaksen 2002; Peake and Manderson 2003). Loss of urinary control strips women of their social rights as adults. Incontinent, they are children again, increasingly wary of the risks of betrayal by their maverick bodies. Fearing exposure of their inability to control their bodies, women limit their social interactions: how often they leave the house, where they shop, what clothes they wear, and how they manage (or avoid) sexual and other intimate relationships. In making sense of this embarrassing but not life-threatening condition, women routinely face contradictions. On the one hand, their incontinence is regarded by women, and their friends and doctors, as a 'normal' part of being female, its incidence explicable if not inevitable because of their personal, embodied history of childbearing and childbirth, menopause and aging. Women with urinary incontinence demonstrate their compliance with gender-appropriate roles, because they have given birth, and for this reason, they have lost continence. Yet in contrast, doctors and the anonymous authors of health education pamphlets often also advise women that their incontinence is due to their deviance – they are overweight, sedentary, have neglected pelvic floor muscles or are generally unfit. Incontinence is presented to women contradictorily as a symbol of their moral worth (having had children) and their moral turpitude (as fat and lazy). Either way, because they are constructed normatively or as deviant, incontinence is represented as normal, part and parcel of being a woman. Given that it is so difficult – socially isolating, logistically complex, sometimes humiliating – to manage urinary incontinence, how much harder is it to manage fecal incontinence (Manderson 2005), or in other ways to manage a transgressive, unpredictable or confronting body?

Ways of Representing

Ideas of the body and its possibilities travel via both old and new media, even when people do not, and medicine, technology, cultural values related to the body, and ideas of self are informed by changes elsewhere. While understandings of the social self constantly shift within the cultural landscape of contemporary English-speaking Australia, there are few differences between Australia and other highly industrialized countries, and the commonalities that flow from globalization lead to similar values and practices everywhere. Developments in medical science and biotechnology, for instance, have led to changes in medical and other clinical practices, and to changes in what is considered socially and medically possible and desirable. These developments and changes are anticipated and described in publications from cyborg politics, philosophy, rehabilitation and disability studies. They are consistent themes, too, in the mass media, in biographical and fictional writing, and in the works of visual artists and commercial and non-commercial filmmakers. Consequently, in this volume, in elucidating the meaning-making that follows accident and illness, and in mapping this onto a cultural canvas, I engage with work from various epistemological and disciplinary strands. Hence this book is eclectic, spanning, synthesizing and engaging with material from the biomedical sciences, social sciences, humanities and the creative arts.

I begin with people's narratives of illness and change. Like public testimonies, ethnographic interviews allow informants to reflect on and hypothesize about their identities and the biological, material, cultural and social circumstances that have shaped them. I use "narrative" to refer to both source and approach, with narrative reconstructions of illness, injury and adaptation providing the empirical flesh of the book. In examining how people seek to come to terms with disabling conditions and/or unorthodox appearance, structure or function following injury or disease, I address what Canguilhem (1991: 31) presents as a menace of incompleteness, a limitation that emerges from within the body. People must accommodate and adapt to their new bodily states, either through dominant or resistant narrative. Most must also address others' discomforts and fears. In many highly disruptive conditions, people seek to come to terms with their condition through conceiving of and reconstructing the event with added spiritual or intellectual meaning (Frankl 1963; Frawley 1997).

Conventional biographic narratives frequently represent corporeal changes in terms of a logical sequence, with a common-sense trajectory leading to the moment of being at the time of telling. The structure of the account and the etiology of conditions may vary depending on a mix of the condition, philosophy and preferred explanatory model – primarily biological or inherited on the one hand, cultural on the other – but the recounting serves to render valid the experience, identity and positioning. In the therapeutic context of a support group, or in individual counseling, or as described in a self-help book, for example, the perceived goal of narration is to establish a sense of validity, an accommodation of the present as a true way of being-in-the-world (Merleau-Ponty 1962). In working through personal history and circumstance, events from the past are positioned in relation to the present, as part of a now inevitable trajectory. In such tales, the emphasis is on the present, with the past retold to establish consistency and a logical outcome or resolution. This approach, enabling the selective telling of biography to fit a dominant and recognizable schema, has been documented for those with changes in identity, for trans- and gay identity, for example, although not necessarily for people who must accommodate physical changes.

Through narrating biography, people find ways to rationalize and accept, tailoring their account so that the present is inevitable and normal. The narrator seeks to claim a sense of coherence; that is, to reject the idea of autobiographical disruption that radically unsettles a sense of self. Each individual story therefore is constructed to bring a phenomenologically real true self into being through a sequence of events and circumstances, including those that relate to health and wellbeing, accident and injury. Most stories, despite their uniqueness, follow a culturally coherent template; they draw on a broad cultural and social environment and so are structured to make intelligible the circumstances of the narrator. Such stories are, of course, adapted and modified over time as circumstances change, as events of the past take on more or less salience, and as perspectives shift. Breast cancer, for instance, may take on a different meaning for family, cultural and medical reasons, depending on whether the person is 35 or 70 years old.

Among the works which inform and reflect cultural trends in the body and identity are the autobiographies of people marginalized by their own corporeality, who have had to address their own corporeal vulnerability, nonconformity and difference. Such written works draw us into the worlds of those whose bodies are archives of trauma or life-threatening disease; indeed, empathetically, into their bodies themselves. Thus Mitchell and Snyder (1997), major US-based cultural theorists of disability, comment on how this literature "provides a glimpse at a unique subjectivity that evolves out of the experience of disability as a physical, cognitive, and social phenomenon" (9), so kneading our understanding of disability, nonconformity and difference. This growing literature includes works of writers who have had congenital health problems. Connie Panzarino (1994), for example, captures both her corporeal and emotional life with muscular dystrophy, balancing her meditations on disability and identity politics with grounded realities: urinating in a polystyrene cup during a street march in New York City, for example. Inga Clendinnen (2000) writes of the onset and tardy diagnosis of active autoimmune hepatitis, of the belly-swelling, bruising and bleeding that continued despite drugs intended to slow her decay, and of her frightening hospitalization and liver transplant. She writes with electric poignancy of her rapid bodily degeneration, with its emotional and mental shock waves as she grappled with her invalidity – as an invalid and as in-valid, the pun Irving Zola (1982) notes – without possible cure or recovery. Nancy Mairs (1987, 1996) writes of the personal loathing, frustration and depression that accompanied her disability and disablement from multiple sclerosis; Jean-Dominique Bauby (1997), in his extraordinary *The Diving Bell and the Butterfly,* as recently translated into film, provides a compelling account of locked-in syndrome. This genre of life stories offers us access to the physical, emotional and social dimensions of disability, the challenge for people to be 'themselves' when they are overpowered by sickness, physical vulnerability and fear, and the difficulty of sustaining relationships with others when the body, the medium for social relationships, is willful.

These non-fictional models are complemented by creative discourses on the body: novels, films, photography, painting, sculpture, performance art, poems and songs, dance and other cultural ephemera: cultural elaborations and interrogations of corporeality. Some of this work requires mediation and translation to those without access to the repertoire of the specific genre; others are explicit and accessible in their methods, content and meaning. In this book, I draw on material from popular culture and the creative arts, the work of independent and commercial film-makers, fiction writers and essayists, visual artworks, art performance, dance and other cultural ephemera: they provide different points of access to the cultural elaboration and interrogation of corporeality. In exploring these cultural products and imagery, I interviewed a number of visual artists, performance artists and actors whose work has been informed by their own illnesses and impairments, and others whose work provocatively critiques and sometimes anticipates developments in science and medical technology.

The visual arts provide powerful exploratory media for alternative narratives of the body and self-perception, esthetics, science and commerce. These creative works are fictions in the everyday meaning of this term – works of the imagination – but they draw on and interpret the real world, reflecting phenomena in ways as relevant and certainly as insightful as non-fictional accounts and scholarly renderings. A significant number of artists, too, have documented their own bodies' histories through their art practice, providing visual texts of diagnosis and treatment, entwined with emotions of fear, despair, hopelessness, anger and conciliation. These works offer fresh ways of thinking about embodiment, disease and disability. Within the world of illness and disease, HIV/AIDS, for instance, stimulated an 'obsession' with the body in art that has been sustained for nearly three decades (Macarow 2006). Although this proliferation of works on HIV and the abject body is relatively recent, it is matched in volume by works on or about breast cancer in the English-speaking world and beyond. Moreover, individual artists have routinely used creative media, including their own and other bodies, to articulate personal crises and contradictions of the body and to document these crises: consider van Gogh's self-portrait of his self-mutilation that has perpetually coupled his art and torment. In so doing, they have pushed bodily boundaries to critique the cultural environment that constructs meanings of the body, its possibilities and demise.

The same understanding applies to film and filmic interpretations or 'readings' of social facts. Commercial films – introduced in the following chapter and revisited later in this volume – capture particularly how the mass media reflects on the body as a site of transgression and possibility, and allows us to trace these ideas as they travel across time and space. Film provides a medium to present data, offering a starting point by which to theorize, represent and analyze habitus and corporeality. In the mass media in its broad manifestations, there has been sustained emphasis – especially from the late 1960s to early 2000s, and less so now – on corporeal change, bodily embellishments, scientific discovery and fantastic possibility. This has been framed by discourses of illness and disability, debates about biotechnology, changing medical practice, policy implications and practical translation, and by reflections and critiques of these developments in biographical and fictional writing, visual art, performance and film, as I illustrate later in this volume.

Other art forms are similarly commentaries on the societies within which they are produced, interrogating their structures and ideologies through specific naturalistic and fanciful images. Each work of art is 'about' the society of which it is part, if not a direct commentary, or about the artist and the audience he or she seeks to address. Indeed, it is hard to imagine a work that could be created outside of society; material culture, environment and discourse provide the artist with the grammar and vocabularies for creativity. While they are, Steven Marcus (1990[1975]:xv) argues, fictions in the everyday meaning of this term, they are connected to the 'real world,' representing and commenting on the same world of which their authors and their audiences are part. Individual artists have routinely used their own and other bodies to articulate personal crises and contradictions *of* the body, pushing bodily boundaries to critique the cultural environment that constructs meanings of the body and its demise.

The visual art I describe allows us to shade in the cultural background in which people come to terms with health crises and adapt to new bodies. We are used to reading the printed text as diachronic and visual art – sculpture, for example – as synchronic. However, visual art has no fewer narrative possibilities than other art forms, even if clearest when presented as a corpus of work, as occurs in a series of paintings by a single artist or as one of a number of items curated for an exhibition. In this book, I have drawn on several exhibitions on the body held in Europe, the U.S. and Australia. Exhibitions are shaped by the authorial hand of the curator, of course, and so explicitly reflect the curator's view, as editors of journals determine the shape of their volumes. But, as Manguel argues (1996), there is more than one way to 'read' a

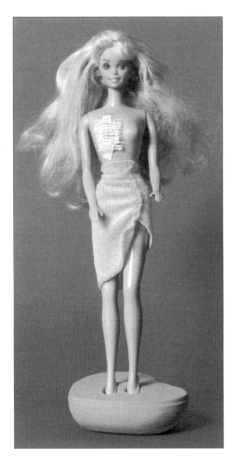

Figure 1.3 Ariela Shavid,
"Barbie Doll," re-worked;
1996. Courtesy of Ariela
Shavid.

collection, and to find new and surprising perspectives in the process. At the same time, many artists are not content to leave the reading-viewing public free to draw its own conclusions, and artists such as Stelarc (see Figure 1.2) and Ju Gosling (Figure 1.4), for example, have taken particular advantage of the Internet to present their own corporeal works and to offer their own exegeses.

Stelarc is an Australian who began as a performance artist in a series of body suspension projects using large fish hooks, undertaken from 1976 in Yokohama and New York (de Groen 1984:98–105; Clark 2003). His website (www.stelarc.vu.edu.au) includes sound, video, VRML, QuicktimeVR and Shockwave files, providing viewers with a summary of the evolution of his work over the past two decades on the limits to corporeality, and

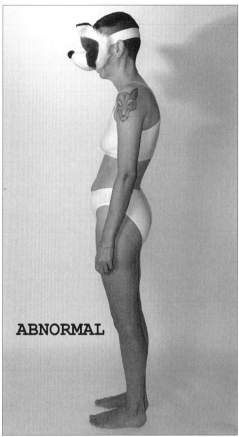

Figure 1.4 Ju Gosling,
Abnormal 1. Lambda print
on aluminum.
© Ju Gosling, aka ju90 2008.

enabling them to 'interview' him virtually about this. Ju Gosling's sensibility draws on her own experience of Scheuermann's Disease. Like Stelarc,
she uses hypermedia and works with film, television and photography and
her own body, through the decorated carapace that supports her spine
(www.ju90.co.uk). The diverse materials that both Gosling and Stelarc
use personalize their experience, but the materials do more than this; they
provide other kinds of narratives and texts, subject to the same kinds of
analyses and inferences and the written or the spoken text. This wider body
of material, primarily but not exclusively from the English-language world,
allows us to theorize further about the context, construction and representation of the body in society and the meanings of intentional, pragmatic
and dysfunctional changes to the body.

Conditions and Methods

At the heart of this book are people who have had little choice in controlling their bodies, surgeries and bodily trajectories. Their experiences, the meanings they give to embodied change, and the measures they take to enhance bodily restitution are set in the cultural landscape of the postmodern English-speaking world in which even greater possibilities of the body are rehearsed. The primary empirical data of *Surface Tensions* are narratives of illness, injury, surgery and recovery, elicited in interviews conducted often on more than one occasion with some one hundred remarkable men and women. In the pages which follow, I explore how people make sense of who they are when the surface of the body is profoundly changed. I ask what occurs when a person experiences a dramatically physical, often very obvious loss, as in the case of the loss of a limb or its functionality. When a woman's sense of being female is so invested in her sexed body, how does she reconstruct 'being feminine' after mastectomy, when surfaces dense with gendered meaning are excised? And how, at the same time, does she make sense of the disease when the challenge to her health is internal and cannot be monitored precisely, even though contemporary technologies extend the clinical gaze to the body's interior? What difference does it make to the self when surfaces are reconstructed and the inner workings of the body are brought to the surface – when elimination must be managed with colostomy bags, for example? And what of the self, when the surface is stable but the inner mechanics of the body change – when, as with a kidney transplant, the body becomes host to an organ vital to survival and once part of someone else? Can the self be whole or undamaged when the body – Janice's "coat to the soul" – has undergone so much change? The interviews on which I draw in this book illustrate how this disorganization is understood and managed by those directly affected.

Morbidity statistics are rarely timely and are often inaccurate. However, the health conditions experienced by the participants in this book are all relatively commonplace, and the surgical procedures are also common; in this respect, the study participants were and are representative of far larger numbers in Australia and elsewhere. People who have had an amputation or have experienced other constraints on physical mobility and muscular control most readily fit into a paradigm of disability, in terms of a body with limited function and in terms of how societies recognize, restrain and accommodate people whose mobility may now depend on an artificial leg or a wheelchair. In Australia, government policy and programs acknowledge the impediments to wellbeing and social inclusion that occur when individuals are isolated due to restricted mobility.

In this volume, I begin my grounded discussion of the body by focusing on people who had had amputations as a result of a workplace, sporting or vehicular accident, from war, or due to disease, usually cancer or complications from diabetes. In Australia, in these times, in a population of some 23 million, there are an estimated 25,000 people with extensive amputations, most beyond retirement age and over 50 percent of whom have lost limbs due to circulatory problems (primarily microvascular complications of diabetes mellitus). Stroke is the second leading cause of death, but is also a major cause of functional difficulty as well as a sign of underlying vascular disease. An estimated 9,000 people live with spinal cord injury, over a quarter from non-traumatic causes. I have also included in my discussions with people with amputations a few people who had lost mobility and full function due to spinal cord injury or stroke.

Others in this book have made transitions from having a chronic disease to living with changes in function and bodily structure, to some degree also with government support. People with stomas, for instance, receive stoma bags free; women with mastectomies are eligible for a subsidy from their state government for initial and replacement breast prostheses, administered either through public hospitals or the Aids and Equipment Program, sufficient to cover the cost of a standard prosthesis. In this volume, I include men and women who had stoma surgery due to colorectal or bladder cancer, inflammatory bowel disease and, less commonly, other bowel, bladder or urethral anomalies that required surgery, and I include women who have had a mastectomy. Some 36,000 people Australia-wide live with a colostomy, ileostomy or urostomy for various reasons, sometimes due to congenital anomalies but more often due to acute or severe chronic disease. Women had had mastectomies because they had been diagnosed with breast cancer, and in a few cases, had opted for mastectomy to prevent its occurrence: one in eleven women experiences breast cancer in her lifetime; slightly fewer than half of these women have a mastectomy as a component of their treatment.

As a fourth category of bodily change, I include men and women with end-stage renal disease who had had kidney transplants, and people who had donated a kidney to a family member. One in seven Australians is at risk of chronic kidney disease, an estimated 2.5 percent of deaths per annum are due to renal failure, and the population requiring dialysis or transplantation is steadily increasing. Additional transplants of heart, lung, liver, pancreas and cornea take place each year.

In summary, I am concerned with the lives of people who have new body parts, replacements or prostheses, or have lost body parts but still perceive them through phantom pain, or who live with parts from others' bodies. Other kinds of cancers and other acute circulatory and muscular-skeletal problems also lead to changes in the surface or the structures of the body and in physical capacity. Stiker's observation that in "us, or around us, the onset of a disability creates a disorganization that is both concrete and social" (1999:3) applies well to these people, who have a stoma, have lost a breast or have had a transplant, as readily as to people who have lost a leg or an arm or are confined to a wheelchair. While the division of body and soul (or body and mind) may be difficult to sustain ethnographically, I share Leder's view of it as an important adaptive response for people seeking restitution following major surgery and body change. Hence, in the title and as a theoretical thread, I use the notion of surface tension. I selected different bodily conditions where there appeared to be surface tension for individuals, usually above the surface, although in the case of transplants, the discordance is largely below the surface. I was interested in commonalities across conditions, where they might be overlooked, and in contrasting different kinds of bodily change to tease out disjunctions between body and self.

The conditions I explore in this book are relatively common: they are prevalent both statistically, such as mastectomy due to breast cancer for instance, and imaginatively, because of media attention given to aspects of the procedures and to the elicitation of public support, as is the case for kidney transplants and requests for donors. These conditions are prevalent at a national level epidemiologically; they are clinically and economically significant; care is often demanding and expensive. They are equally important socially and personally: their occurrence, diagnosis, management and prognosis have great significance for those directly affected, and for their families, because of how they impact functional ability, independence, autonomy and self-identity. Yet the conditions, and the existential crises that they invoke, have attracted little interest from social scientists. Social and health psychology is a partial exception, with a voluminous literature on conditions such as breast cancer. Anthropologists, however, have contributed little, arguably because of our emphasis on community and context rather than care and the clinical domain.

Because of the social significance of particular clinical conditions, my recruitment of participants was defined by outcome; their categorical positioning is, therefore, an artifact of biomedicine. Not surprisingly, people transgressed these strict diagnostic categories. Many participants, like Perdita, had complicated histories of chronic illness and surgery, and those whom I interviewed for one condition often experienced and lived with several – multiple cancers, multiple body losses, multiple surgeries: colostomy and urostomy, for example, mastectomy and ileostomy, spinal cord injury, urostomy and renal failure, amputation and stroke, and so on. Hence their stories of personal adaptation, resilience, social support, re-creation of character and repositioning of self are, as might be expected, always noisier and more complicated than a medical diagnosis would suggest.

My recruitment of people with specific medical histories was also practical. Medical, health and ancillary services in Australia are intended to help people by providing them with practical links and avenues for support from rehabilitation services, consumer associations, help-groups and the like. These associations provide a mechanism for health providers to get information to consumers, and for consumers – clients, patients – to share their experiences and their strategies in managing aspects of their personal, social and physical lives. I was introduced by social workers to people with end-stage renal disease. Personal referrals and chance introductions also steered me to potential participants. Other people found me. One letter began, "I am writing to you to ask to be included in the study. You will recall that we met in 1989." Another: "I was checking out your website to enroll in a course and I noticed that you are doing a study that has personal relevance to me." These interviews were supplemented with letters, self-taped reflections, and questionnaire returns from an additional fifty-five people I was unable to meet in person, who wished even so to provide me with an account of their accommodation to the surgical and medical disruptions in their lives.

These methods of recruitment and collection of information took advantage of various technologies and networks – the distribution of supplies and information by the government to individuals with certain conditions, membership of consumer associations, the use of the Internet and email as well as print media, and individuals' own familiarity with research and their wish to be part of it. People wanted their stories heard and told (Warren, Markovic, Manderson 2006). In supplementing this material, and in testing my ideas, I participated in, addressed and observed meetings of consumer associations, professional associations and support groups, using these fora to recruit new participants and to test my own ideas and interpretations. I analyzed newsletters produced by consumer groups, published and circulated reports, web pages of individuals and groups, and newspaper accounts: this primary literature is voluminous. And as my ideas took shape, I tested them in other research projects. The core data in this book, therefore, are supplemented with interviews and questionnaire data from an additional 300 participants from other studies on lower-limb amputation, diabetes, gynecological illness and a range of chronic and degenerative conditions.

Strangers may be entirely unaware of the conditions of many of these people, and only those who rely on wheelchairs would be included as a matter of course in a conventional social or medical model of disability. Nor would individuals so affected necessarily embrace an identity of disability, despite that their conditions impact their everyday lives. Even so, understandings of disability are invaluable in assisting our understanding of how individuals (and their families) adjust to the engineering detours and the practical management of their bodies. Life-saving surgery and rehabilitation programs transfer these men and women from the world of medical drama and incapacity to a world of negotiable and variable disability, shaped by the physical, social and cultural environment. Support groups, family crises and personal attitudes to the body and its (missing) parts all contribute to perceptions of embodied difference and adaptation.

Storytelling of the Making of the Self

The discourses around body/mind distinctions emphasize that the idea of the individual – I, the self, counter-positioned against others – is culturally variable, and suppositions about and expressions of individuality are themselves culturally constructed. My task as author has been to gather the common threads of meaning from these individual accounts, and to relate these to the cultural context of English-speaking Australians.

For people who deal with confronting assaults on and changes to the body, the shared story has a further role, in establishing with others commonality of experience and therefore normality, composing for each person a picture of a normal way of being with embodied change. This is true for individuals who tell their stories in a support group, by writing a letter to a newsletter, or by posting a commentary on a website, or who share their experience with an anthropologist (Warren, Markovic and Manderson 2006). Through narration, the storyteller reaches out to others, and here, there is resistance: the normal 'ideal' is disrupted as people establish the actual, expected and lived experiences of their own bodily conditions, and the commonality of their experiences with the experiences of others. Normal is a relative concept: individuals act in ways that are normal for them. The self offers its own benchmarks, and people exercise measures of freedom to personalize their own accounts of illness, disease or injury, and adaptation to change, moving discursively between their own circumstances and the larger order of things. Narratives therefore work to establish the personal coherence of biography in the context of social and cultural forces, and the individual's position within society and in relation to others. Such factors include whether individuals are partnered or not at the time of their accident or illness, whether they can afford the time and money to pursue a particular course of treatment, and whether they choose or are able to choose to join a support group that might contribute to meaning-making through shared narratives of illness and outcome. As already noted, the primary data are extensive interviews with individuals who have lived through medical crises and surgical resolutions, with various repercussions on structure and function, body image, personhood, gender and sexuality. Their accounts of illness and adaptation clarify questions of body boundaries and the self. In conducting the interviews, I encouraged participants to tell their own story, maintaining flexibility so that they might provide full and meaningful accounts of events and their significance, and theorize about these in ways that are not part of conventional everyday discourse. While the bare bones of the history of illness or injury and surgery are retold, fuller reflections are rarely discussed beyond the crises of the moment. The interviews allowed informants to reflect on and hypothesize about their identities and the biological, material and social circumstances that shaped them, but as always, accounts are shaped by the interactions of the interviewer and interviewee (Manderson, Bennett, Andajani-Sutjahjo 2006). Consequently, the interaction has a formative effect; events crystallize in the process of recounting. Each storyteller reconstructed his or her biography, recalling, rehearsing, interpreting and redefining to bring together past and present, to create a "coherent sense of self-identity" and narrative unity (Benhabib 1992). Through the narrative accommodation to a condition or state of being, transforming social identity through resistance to dominant ideology, disruptions are given purpose and new identities are forged.

I began this book with Perdita's story. Not all participants had such extensive medical histories, nor were they as self-reflective as Perdita. All had opinions about their bodily histories, however, and about the impact of surgery on their own lives and their personal relationships. People act in ways that are normal for others like themselves and are comprehensible to others who are unlike them. As they offer their own interpretive frameworks and theories, contemporary discourse and history remain the reference point. Individual stories are intelligible because of their consistency within given contexts, and the institutions, ideologies and structures of a given cultural, political and economic setting all shape the meanings of embodied change and possible trajectories and outcomes. Hence my interest in this work of capturing the broad social and cultural environment, including films, literature, visual art, advertising and everyday body practices that inform people's story telling of their bodies and provide them with a contemporary logic to their state of being. These provide people with templates or frameworks to adjust, find meaning, and move forward.

Lingis (1994) has claimed that the relationship between interviewer and interviewee, or researcher and interlocutor, is always inherently uneven, one inevitably silenced by the other: "When the other is there and able to speak himself or herself, he or she listens to the thoughts one formulates for him or her, and assents to them or contests them or withdraws from them into the silence from which he or she came. One only speaks for others when they are silent or silenced. And to speak for others is to silence oneself" (1994:ix). But this perspective assumes immutable polarity in conducting research, and ignores the variability that occurs from one interview to the next. I prefer to see relationships in ethnography and other kinds of social research as negotiated; the descriptive and analytic voice in the final text reflects this stance. The men and women who contributed to this book make sense of their bodily interruptions, disruptions and surgeries in the context of their own lives. They were well aware that this was so; several early in interviews took control of the interaction and told me the story they wanted to tell, weaving a narrative around the events that they considered to be core to their identity and explaining the specific and unique ways in which assaults to their health worried at or reinforced this identity.

To the extent that I draw out stories of embodied lives from my research participants, however, my approach shares conceptual ground with narrative epistemology. Narrative approaches within anthropology and cognate fields (social psychology, sociology, social linguistics) pay particular attention to the structure and content of the stories, as each person situates his or her own history and yet draws on and creates a culturally logical reality. Like other kinds of narratives, accounts of illness or injury attend to the patterns and disruptions in a person's life; these are transformed in the storytelling into events with purpose. There are many ways to tell a story and many stories can be told. We all tell tales of who we are for public consumption, twisting our accounts to fit the presumed interests of a given audience, and we tell private stories with intimates, varying the details as we lay bare our 'real' selves. Moments of drama and joy are injected into such accounts, not as inexplicable detours, but as the hills and vales of a singular trajectory. People whose lives detour dramatically draw upon tropes and clichés – *getting in touch with yourself, finding out who you really are, getting real* – to explain the importance to them of narrative coherence, to explain their positioning to others, to make sense of their deviance from social expectation, and to account for the decisions that informed the direction of their lives. They must retell their stories to make sense of the present (Frank 1995).

The Body of the Text

In chapter 2, I provide a historic backdrop to the present setting in which people practice and think about their bodies. This includes reflecting on changes in medical and surgical practice, including early experimental work and advanced surgical techniques and transplants, and the possibilities rehearsed with developments in the fields of immunology and immunotherapy, genetics, microsurgery and pharmacology. These developments are not regarded in contemporary society without ambivalence.

Chapters 3 to 6 are built around interviews with men and women who have had to deal with acquired external or internal physical impairments and corporeal change, which, as noted, include amputation or loss of function, a stoma, mastectomy and transplant. In chapter 3, I discuss physical difference as experienced by men and women who have lost the use of their limbs as a result of an accident or from a stroke, or who have lost a limb from an industrial, vehicular or war-related accident or a medical condition – diabetic neuropathy and infection, gangrene from atherosclerosis, or cancer. An amputation or bodily immobility is a blatant example of a body unable to be controlled; as Lennard Davis (1995:12) notes, "disability is a specular moment." The stump or lifeless limb is constant evidence of decay or damage too gross, too excessive, to be repaired or restored. Subsequently, the individual must learn to negotiate with lack – walking with a prosthetic leg or using a wheelchair, using various other aids to enable independent living, or relying on others for daily practicalities. Life-long dependency, varying according to the severity of loss of function and the social environment, can place an adult perpetually in the position of child, and people who have experienced major changes in physical ability and body function due to accident or illness, becoming wheelchair bound, for instance, lose a range of societal rights conferred on able-bodied adults. People with amputation frequently draw on a discourse of normality to resist the disempowerment that is inevitable with infantilization. Their insistence on normalcy, described in this chapter, illustrates how such surface changes to the body impact upon social membership. In demonstrating normalcy, men and women draw on normative conventions – those associated with femininity for women, masculinity for men – to accentuate gender normativity. Men do, and women are. I conclude this chapter with an example of resistance, and the risks that people take when they choose to embrace rather than disguise their bodily selves.

In chapter 4, I turn to the experiences of men and women who have lost continence and have required stoma surgery to eliminate body waste. One of the earliest tasks of a child is to master the etiquette of continence: to adopt in a near-automatic manner control over invisible muscles to contain body waste – a perfect example of habitus to evacuate in the right place, to maintain discretion over such functions, and to observe cultural codes of decorum. Toilet training takes precedence over virtually all behaviors other than the first bodily tasks of ingestion, walking and talking – the basic survival skills of communication and locomotion. In this chapter, I explore how men and women adjust to a stoma and adapt to the mechanical care of bowel or bladder. Here the surface tension relates to surgical changes to body structure and function. With a colostomy or ileostomy, this includes the removal of anus and rectum, the loss of the sphincter (and so the loss of control of the timing of defecation), the diversion of the colon to the surface of the belly, and the manual removal of feces collected in a bag. Sarbin (1997: 67) has argued that people construct an identity by drawing on stories that provide the plot structures for self-narrative (see also Frank 1995). They are selective, however, in constructing their identities, shaping their biography so that the present is the most obvious, best possible and desirable outcome. This is difficult to do when the present is personally undesired and socially undesirable.

People with stomas harness a discourse of normalcy, but for many, this is difficult to sustain when the normal body is out of control in either public or private settings. As I illustrate, people negotiate their body surface in space, particularly in intimate contexts where they can literally and metaphorically come unstuck (Manderson 2005).

Gender is a starting point of individual construction and re-construction of the self. Cultural norms of persons as social actors also shape social reactions and so predict the social impact of disease or accident. Loss of body parts, functions and appearance have negative valence. In chapter 5, I explore the experiences of women who have lost a breast or both breasts, either from breast cancer or because the risk of developing cancer was so great that they had a prophylactic mastectomy. Here, I illustrate how deeply gender is embedded in the flesh: breasts are the quintessential gender surface. Drawing on interview data and the work of visual artists with breast cancer, I illustrate how losing a breast cuts into and away at a woman's sense of being female and feminine, her self-confidence and assurance, regardless of her ability to dismiss the importance of breasts as a societal superficiality. Not all women mourned the loss of their breasts – a few were sanguine – but most women were uncomfortable with their bodies, scarred and concave, post-surgery. As with men and women with stoma, women who had had mastectomies learned a new manner of embodiment, dressing, displaying and protecting their chests and/or prosthetic breasts to minimize psychological rather than physical discomfort. The interview data are framed by my discussion of the art of both Melissa Jane Ades and Ariela Shavid, who represent visually their experiences of the disease, its treatment, and the tensions between personal loss and societal values.

Men and women who have transplants have a particular need to separate their physical and social self, body and soul, to maintain a sense of self and an understanding of personal continuity following changes in corporeality. The context of transplant surgery is one of scientific advancement and heroic medicine, but also of cultural anxieties about bodily substance, individual consubstantiality, the nature of creation and being, the provenance of body parts, and the ethics of experimentation. A number of scholars have written about the ethical tensions of transplantation, including the problematic definition of brain death, shifting attitudes towards life support, and an apparently incessant demand for body parts, reflected in allegations of the kidnapping and murder of people from the poorest countries in the world to 'harvest' and sell organs, and the sale of 'spare parts' by those who are too poor to meet their own subsistence needs. But those who give and receive organs are relatively absent in these accounts. In chapter 6, I consider the embodied experiences of men and women with end-stage renal disease who require dialysis, and the unique surface tensions that exist as they rely on technology to do the work of an inner organ. In the context of kidney transplants, I then discuss the centrality of the social body: how people who choose to give or receive a kidney feel about the donor or the context of life and death when the kidney is from a cadaver, and contemplate the genesis of the organ and the component parts of the physical body that contribute to their being.

In chapter 7, I return to general cultural concerns about medicine and sciences of the body, particularly as reflected and debated in popular film. I see in contemporary drama and science fiction the revisiting of questions about the nature of the self, at the same time as film makers conjure up for viewers the technical capacities of modern societies and other imagined ways of embodied being. I discuss also the work of visual artists, industrial designers and performers who are critical of these developments. The technical advantages to individuals are countered by fears of medicine out-of-hand, excesses of surgery and biological experiment. Here ethical issues and fancy often collide – a hand with a life of its own or a humanoid with razor digits undermining or emphasizing questions of the direction, possibility and desirability of various scientific experiments, xenotransplantation and cloning. I conclude by revisiting what I see as core features of the contemporary experience of embodiment – the nature of gender and the construction of normalcy. These I consider to be adaptive strategies for men and women whose bodies straddle the states of sickness and wellbeing.

Contemporary concerns about the ethics and eugenic implications of stem-cell research, new reproductive technologies and reproduction in post-menopausal women, or vanity procedures to reduce signs of aging, are rarely debated in the context also of the exigencies of threatened life or the disempowerment that flows from certain impairment. The debates rarely take account of the individual meanings or lived experiences of chronic illness or disability. Contemporary theories of the body and society similarly are often aloof from ordinary bodies and bodily experiences, the mundane management of bodily processes and body waste. Together, the chapters offer an appreciation of the everyday complexities for people who must work with their bodies.

In writing of surface tensions of the body and the shock waves that extend to individual selves, I consider how people make meaning from being both "strange and a stranger" in their own eyes and in the eyes of others (Stiker 1999:8). "No investigation has the right to present its results as the totality, as complete," Stiker (2) wrote a decade ago; this work is no exception. Social investigations such as this work aim to lift the covers off social life, to open to light phenomena not yet exposed, described or interrogated, to unsettle orthodoxy and to reinterpret conventional wisdom. Each story is unique, yet patterns emerge, too, from the stories people tell. They have a cultural consistency. While I ask in relation to scientific experiment, Is the body obsolete?, I conclude by requiring that we remain sensitive to the needs of those whose bodies are at the center of these debates and whose lives often depend on these technologies.

2 🪶

Our Cyborg Selves, and Other Modern Tales

My mother is the last person on the day's list for one of the most common surgeries performed worldwide: small incision surgery to remove a cataract that obscures her vision and to replace the natural lens with an artificial one. After mild local anesthesia, a small cut is made above her iris; the cataract is broken up with ultrasonic vibrations, and the debris is removed by suction through the opening. A foldable acrylic intraocular lens is inserted through the incision, and once in the lens capsular bag, it opens out to full size. Ninety minutes later, a patch over one eye, her glasses unevenly atop, using a light-weight walking frame to steady her gait, she walks through the door of the hospital to go home. Less than twenty-four hours later, the bandage has been removed and she begins seeing the world more brightly and clearly. A few years later, the surgery is repeated to redress my rapid loss of vision: my cataractic lenses are replaced, five days apart; it takes seven minutes and minimal anesthesia to undertake the surgery. I have a cup of tea when I come to, and catch the train home afterwards; the morning after, I awake to discover the brilliance of white.

My mother's cataract surgery was one of a series of common surgeries, calendar points of her later years. Hip-replacement for osteoarthritis, the bone and cartilage of the upper end of the femur and the acetabulum replaced with a new ceramic ball and socket, bringing to an end the excruciating pain that had dominated her daily life and woken her each time she turned at night. Surgery corrects structural deformity of a hammer toe that had lead to painful lesions, difficulties with footwear and walking; the joints are realigned with fine stainless steel, and she regains the mobility that had almost disappeared. Around the house, now even the walking stick is unnecessary. Light weight aluminum pick-up reachers of different lengths extend her arms, saving her from stooping to pick up the smallest item that falls from bench to floor. Hip replacement, artificial

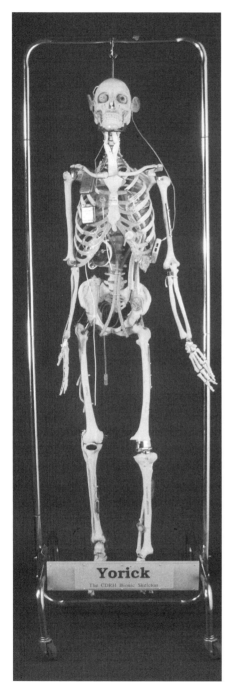

lens, dental crowns, fillings and plate, glasses, four-point and single point walking sticks, a static frame and a four-wheel walking frame with seat, carry-basket and press-down brakes … My mother is a cyborg.

These kinds of surgeries and everyday interfaces with technology evoked Donna Haraway's (1991:179) reflections on the fusion of the technological and organic; twenty years on, they are commonplace for many if not most people in high income countries. Yet the everyday procedures and appliances that have produced cyborg bodies have long histories. Cataract surgery, for instance, took place from the fifth century BC, was mentioned in Sanskrit manuscripts from this time, and was described both in the Code of Hammurabi (1750 BC) and by Celsus in *De Medicinae* in 29 AD. Gaby Wood (2002:41–42) claims that one of Louis XV's chief surgeons, La Peyronie, performed cataract operations, and already by

Figure 2.1 *Yorick, the bionic skeleton;* **2003.** Courtesy of the Food and Drug Administration, U.S. Department of Health and Human Services; Smithsonian Institution National Museum of American History, Kenneth E. Behring Center.

the mid eighteenth century in Britain and France, cataracts were extracted fundamentally as they are today. Intraocular lenses were developed in 1949, and since then the primary scientific advance has been simply the development of a softer acrylic lens, which can be folded into the eye through a minute incision at the edge of the sclera or cornea, so obviating the need for suture. Worldwide today, an estimated 8 million people have cataract surgery, often conducted by paramedics, to restore or improve their vision. Cybervision is routine and normal.

Hip replacement is less common than cataract surgery globally because of the lower prevalence of osteoarthritis, the primary reason for the surgery, and because of varied access to surgery. Even so, the procedure is one of the most common in industrialized countries where health insurance is available and the prosthetic affordable, and is an increasingly common reason for international medically-related travel. Hip, knee and other joint replacements have risen dramatically over the past decade worldwide. Australia's national joint replacement registry, which captures most if not all surgeries in the country, indicates that hip replacement rose from 600 in 1999 and 5,800 in 2000 to 32,400 in 2008; knee replacement surgery increased even more quickly from 500 in 1999 and 5,500 in 2000 to 39,100 in 2008 and is still increasing. For most people in this country, pain in a joint is a presage of surgery; the question is simply one of timing. Replacement surgery on shoulders, elbows, wrists, ankles and the spine, as soon as technically possible, also began to rise in incidence.

But again, these are not procedures entirely new to the late twentieth and early twenty-first century. Experimental surgery for hip replacement, using gold and ivory, dates from the late 1800s, and by the 1920s, glass, then plastic and stainless steel, were being used to replace the femoral head. By 1961, current surgical techniques had been developed to replace an arthritic hip joint with a metal ball and polyethylene plastic socket. More recent modifications and refinements relate primarily to the materials used – the stem, ball and socket using combinations of plastic, cobalt, chromium and titanium – and to the variable outcomes of different femoral and acetabular components to support osteointegration, that is, the merging of the artificial with natural bone. And foot surgery is almost as common as knee and hip arthroplasty, and common deformities such as hammer toe, claw toe and mallet toe, exacerbated if not caused by fashion footwear, all requiring surgical correction. By the early twenty-first century, therefore, orthopedic surgery had become mundane in terms of science and technology because of the relative straightforwardness of the procedures and so their success rates. With its dramatically increased prevalence, such surgery had also become mundane in everyday terms, the expected means by which to remove or reduce pain and immobility and restore wellbeing and physical capacity. And while for a period following surgery, a patient must slowly gain agility, flexion and strength, the incorporation of the prosthesis – the integration of artificial parts into the body – is largely muted, phenomenologically absent in Leder's terms.

Locality and socio-economic status strongly predict who has surgery and when they have it, as well as the quality of the prostheses. Gender, however, influences the kinds of cyborgs that men and women become. Women predominate as patients for hip replacements for osteoarthritis. Not surprisingly, they also predominate for foot surgery, crippled over time by wearing narrow or confining footwear with increased heel height. For cataract surgery, too, women predominate, although as a simple artifact of their greater longevity; while 50 percent of people develop cataracts by the age of 60, 100 percent have done so by the age of 80 (Hammond 2001). In Australia, my mother's transmogrification as a cyborg is typical of women of her age and social background. She and her friends and relatives are not alone, however. Routine questionnaires are now administered to all people prior to an MRI, checking for a wide range of corrective, protective and cosmetic products – a hip or knee replacement, a pacemaker, an implanted drug infusion device, metal pins, plates or screws, a neurostimulator, embolization coil, intraventricular shunt, renal shunt or wire sutures, an IUD, body piercing jewelry or tattooed eyelids, or other. Any foreign body might interfere with imaging. The questions and the use of technical language to describe the procedures and techniques point to the common-place nature of such surgery within society. The demand for them far exceeds the ability of the public health system to meet it; for publicly funded 'elective' surgery, delays are routine, symptomatic of inequities in medical services and hospital care.

The predominant reasons for surgical augmentation and replacement in Australia and other industrialized countries highlight that most modern cyborgs are elderly. Yet the cultural imaginary of the cyborg as futuristic and young prevails. And as a result, older people are often overlooked in the consideration of corrective surgery and debates about disability. The social and economic impact of various health conditions, and the structural disadvantages and exclusion that occur in consequence, separate those with life-long or major acquired disabilities and those who have lost function with age. Disability is so normalized with old age as to lose any political import. Being able-bodied, however, is a temporary thing, illusive and elusory. Almost all of us, if we live long enough, will lose sensory acuity, mobility and function. Older people are vulnerable to commercial forces – products and procedures, unguents and embrocations, tonics and laser techniques – that promise to rejuvenate and beautify. Body parts that function inadequately or break down, as well as bodies that fail for reasons of birth or disease to meet the functional and esthetic values of a given place and time, are increasingly objects of intense market competition as technology and surgery move from corrective or rehabilitative to cosmetic purpose, even if the multiple purposes interlace.

Take eyes, for example. Glasses, Manguel (1996:291) suggests, are "eyes that poor-sighted readers can pull off and put on at will. They are a detachable function of a body." Hand-held magnifying glasses were used well before the contemporary era, probably with the accidental discovery of magnification through glass. The first wearable eye glasses date only from the late thirteenth century in Italy, as depicted in art works of St. Lucy and St. Jerome from this time, and their documented use by monks

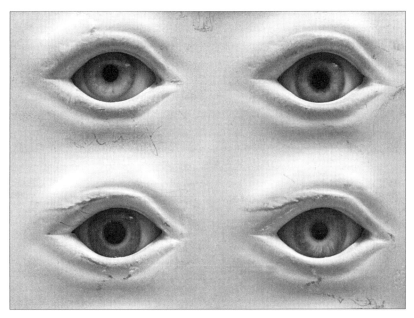

Figure 2.2 Rudolf Martin, *Glass eyes in a tin box, Germany;* late nineteenth century. Glass/aluminum/tin/wood/paint. Photograph by Sotha Bourn. Courtesy of Powerhouse Museum, Sydney.

and others whose eyesight was compromised by close work requiring continual clear vision. The bifocal lens was invented in 1784 by Benjamin Franklin; the contact lens by Adolf Flick in 1887. Glasses have long been commonplace. Again, in recent years, many in wealthier settings have made the transition from artificial lens to laser surgery to correct mild to moderate myopia, and a growing clientele now opts for the latest surgical techniques for severe myopia, with contact lenses implanted under the cornea to maximize correction. Hence a range of tools and devices, archaic and modern, external to and extensions of the body, deal with eye problems: white canes and walking sticks, seeing-eye (guide) dogs, braille, audio-recorded books, magnifying glasses, telescopes, binoculars, 3D glasses, glass eyes, glasses with single, bifocal, trifocal, and graded lenses, shaded, colored and light sensitive tints; corrective and cosmetic contact lenses, hard lenses, soft lenses, disposable lenses; laser surgery for myopia, astigmatism and glaucoma; cataract surgery and lens implants; blepharoplasty (eyelid surgery); talking equipment (talking bathroom scales, for example, enabling the blind as well as the sighted surveillance of their bodies); text-to-speech software to allow people with vision impairment to 'read' with a computer. As these techniques and interventions have gained sophistication, effectiveness, durability and affordability, the market has shifted from the therapeutic and prosthetic to the esthetic, explaining the extraordinary market of fashion frames, disposable and colored contact lenses. And so to eye candy, contact lenses of fanciful color and iris design. The intention is not to minimize difference while overcoming physical impediments that inhibit social activity, but rather, perversely, through the attention-drawing mechanism of the party eye, the wearer accentuates her normalcy and her (sexual) desirability. Women (and men) who require major corrective surgery and/or must wear thick optical lenses to negotiate their own bodies through space do not have the liberty to don cats' eyes contact lenses or match their iris with their clothes. At the same time, predictably, in line with resistance to medicalization and ideological commitment to the natural (Radcliffe-Richards 1982), alternative resources for improved vision are marketed. One New York clinic – and there are hundreds like it in any cosmopolitan center – offers clients eye-care without drugs or surgery for both old-fashioned eye problems (eyestrain, double vision, lazy eyes, crossed eyes) and a host of postmodern culture-specific syndromes and neuroses – computer visual distress, post-traumatic vision syndrome, attention deficit disorder, learning related vision problems, and so on. And to these, we should add also pharmaceutical products and cosmetics: eye drops, creams, kohl, mascara. In terms of cosmetics and correction, the eyes have it.

With less gimmickry but no fewer pecuniary gains for its specialists, consider, too, the advances in dental management and technology: dentures, fillings, crowns, braces and bands (plain and colored) and dental implants, leading to a growing number of 'oral implantologists' and an expanding dental tourist market in newly industrializing countries and the politico-economic south. This is only part of a market that has expanded dramatically in economic value. Instant tooth whitening through porcelain resurfacing and gold caps for ostentatious display rather than caries prevention are one end of a market that in a commercial pharmacy or drug store is as banal as tooth picks, flosses, pastes and powders to prevent decay, discoloration and mouth odor, in order to maintain social relationships and dental and gum health. Here, it is difficult to segregate public health and commercial gains: to encourage people to follow the regimens of dental hygiene, capitalist enterprises have played on personal and social insecurities.

As for eyes and teeth, so for ears. The outer ear is already well decorated, for men and women in this present time, with earrings, cuffs and studs. But substantial advances have been made, too, since the first trumpets and hearing aids to augment sound. Today a person might, depending on the degree and location of impairment, choose from systems that use analogue or digital sound processing. The latter are encoded to facilitate measurement and reproduction of pitch and volume: they vary from the

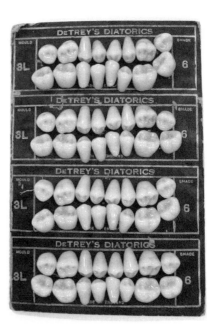

Figure 2.3 Set of porcelain artificial teeth. Made for the Amalgamated Dental Co. Ltd., London, England by Detrey's Diatorics. Used at the Lakeside Hospital, a mental health hospital, located in Ballarat, Australia; 1925. Courtesy of the Museum Victoria.

minute Completely-In-the-Canal (CIC) instruments located well in the ear canal, larger In-the-Canal (ITC) and In-the-Ear (ITE) instruments to meet a wider range of hearing losses, accommodating larger sound amplifiers and features such as a telephone switch, to the robust behind-the-ear aids available in various colors and shapes. These are supplemented by other assistive technologies: telephone and personal television amplifiers, text telephones, personal communicators, alert devices, group listening devices. The most intrusive of these is the cochlear implant, developed in the twentieth century and heralded as the ultimate solution to assist people who were profoundly deaf to hear.

Again, although its sophisticated technology suggests its recency, the development of the multi-electrode 'bionic ear' dates from experiments conducted in Italy in 1790 with frogs, and in 1800, by applying electrical stimuli to the auditory nerves of humans. When its Australian inventor Grahame Clarke was undertaking research in the 1960s and 1970s, therefore, he was building on work from a number of different centers in Europe in particular. The introduction of the cochlear implant generated considerable controversy, related in part to cost and access, but in part, importantly, to the supposition that people who could be so assisted would want to and should take advantage of the technology (see Figure 2.4). Those who have challenged this supposition, including many within the Deaf community, have regarded cochlear implants as a technology that threatens cultural integrity, potentially marginalizing people who for physiological, cultural, financial or other reasons cannot or chose not to use a hearing aid, while diluting efforts by the Deaf to gain respect and diversity in communication modes and cultural style (Davis 1995; Davidson 2008). Popular esthetics prescribe the normal body and normal body functions, and in doing so, mandate the use of prosthetics with cosmetic as well as functional appeal to 'normalize' people in an ableist world.

Arguments against technological innovation that blur the distinctions between hearing aids, cochlear implants, and computerized virtual reality, for instance, fail to differentiate need and want, survival and indulgence. This blurring occurs in various fields of medical science, technology, and surgical correction and enhancement, often with the effect of questioning the motivation of the person who is directly affected, who has sought out the intervention for a complex mix of reasons. Notwithstanding the pervasiveness of ideologies of normalcy and normal function, the technologies that have developed in line with other

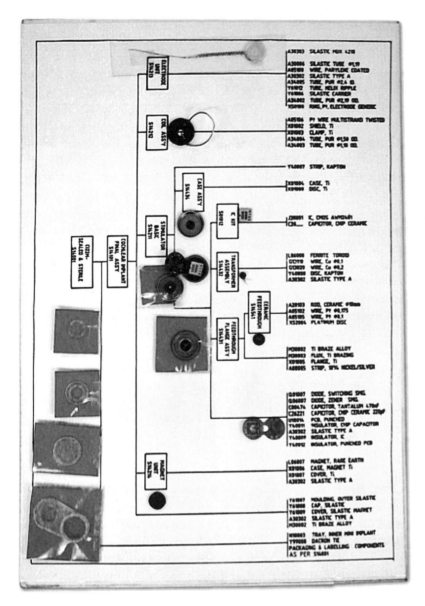

Figure 2.4 Implant components, cochlear implant. Metal/silicone/paper. **Cochlear Pty Ltd, Australia; 1991.** Courtesy of Cochlear 2011 Collection: Powerhouse Museum, Sydney.

advances in biomechanics, neurophysiology, immunology, pharmacology and surgery enable many people with diverse debilitating conditions to enjoy an active, extended and enhanced life. The pacemaker is one example of an exquisite technology, first developed as an external fixture in 1932 and now placed internally, and so largely out of mind. Operated by a lithium battery, it intervenes and takes over to correct abnormally slow or irregular heartbeat, preventing symptoms such as dizziness, extreme fatigue, shortness of breath, or fainting spells that inhibit everyday living activities and may result in heart failure and death. The memory in the pacemaker, too, provides the cardiologist with a record of the heart's workings over the previous year, chronicling the occasions when the pacemaker took over and corrected impeded natural heart function. It is difficult to characterize the introduction and wide use of the pacemaker as evidence of run-away technology and heroic medicine. Other new technologies are simply lighter and more efficient for those who use them, and while they are sometimes more esthetically pleasing, they do not necessarily dilute the negative connotations and stereotypes associated with disability. Although the visible use of assistive technologies produces stigma and with it, its own economic and social exclusion, without these technologies, many people are excluded absolutely.

Querying Normalcy

> *What might appear as a wholesale movement towards the narcissistic cultivation of bodily appearance is in fact an expression of a concern lying much deeper actively to "construct" and control the body. (Giddens 1991:7)*

Culture and biology interlace, and it is difficult to imagine a body pre-existent of culture or independent of its social moorings. "Palpable and visible, the body's contours, anatomical features, processes, movements, and expressions" (Urla and Terry 1995:6) are now given cultural meaning: culture makes value judgments about different types of bodies, tying moral worth to beauty, fitness and conformity and assuming that divergence in form and appearance reflects character flaws. Much of our analysis of the normal and the pathological, the normative and transgressive, owes a debt to the work of Canguilhem. As he notes (1994), in the biological sciences, as in mathematics, the abnormal is defined in relation to deviation from the mean rather than the normal being defined in relation to its proximity to the ideal. Insofar as both the usual or habitual and the ideal merge in social understandings of the normal, there is also considerable ambiguity and space for resistance, as reflected in disability activism and in the idea of the freak (Garland-Thomson 1996;1997a), but also because of changes in technical knowledge and practice. While the interrogation and challenges of cultural constructions of the body, normalcy and deviance are an important project, it is also important, for reasons of social justice, to understand the impact of these constructions of bodies for those who live with 'deviant' bodies. A key purpose of this book is to illustrate how people negotiate bodily appearance and representation to minimize the impact of differences of normal and deviant, to live 'normally' regardless of bodily diversity or (culturally defined) deviation, and to work with bodies that inhibit mobility, function and action.

Body identity can be problematic when people's bodies deviate from cultural norms. Under conditions of modernity, as Giddens (1991) argued two decades ago, self-identity is an organized endeavor, rehearsed and delivered reflexively. In contemporary industrialized societies and increasingly in newly industrializing societies, where people have access to diverse goods and services and autonomy over their own resources, lifestyle and the body itself are a constituent part of the project of identity building, reflecting and informing its expression. This project of identity building includes body maintenance, diet, fitness and dress, decisions about kinds of health care, procedures adopted to maintain good health, the choice of self-presentation, residence, organization of activities, employment and personal life. For many these are increasingly ordinary actions, choices and expenditures for those able to pay, contrasting with the inability of others, who for economic reasons especially have no choice in body management and care. Vast discrepancies within and between cultures and societies, and as a result of structural vulnerabilities and inequalities, impede health and tamper with the ability of people to manage bodily ailments and anomalies. Gender, ethnicity, race and age interact with and compound class position, too; all are barriers to choice. Waiting lists for surgical procedures instantiate these inequalities. Those who are poor and who rely on public hospital services, often run down and understaffed, may wait years (as occurs for hip replacement), and may be rejected for reasons such as (over)weight and general health status. Disability also strips people of choice; and as I shall illustrate, people who have experienced catastrophic bodily change have far less opportunity to control the direction and flow of their lives. Poverty, obesity, lack of mobility, and associated health problems coincide. People with private health insurance, on the other hand, depending on their disposable income, may face relatively little delay.

A number of writers, scholarly and creative, have documented how people with physical disabilities have embraced the technologies of the cyborg body, using prosthetic enhancements to access the worlds of the able-bodied. The attraction for both elderly and younger people to embrace technologies, surgical procedures and pharmaceuticals as they become safely available and relatively affordable is simply to be able to live a well enough, free enough life. Surgery, rehabilitative medicine, prostheses and orthoses, and various other assistive devices – voice-recognition software, enlarged dial pads on phones, for instance – are designed to address the most immediate, physical aspects of disability, maximizing individual functions such as locomotion and personal care of the body, and minimizing the stigma directed at and internalized by people who are, by appearance, 'Other.' Unlike various cosmetic surgical procedures, these measures are rarely radical or gratuitous; rather, while acknowledging ableist majority values and institutions, they are measures that help shape the trajectories of people's lives. They consequently draw attention to the profound and mundane ways in which bodies can interfere with everyday living.

Consider the walking frame, unmodified in design or function for centuries. Hieronymous Bosch, in his painting Christ Child with a Walking Frame, depicts the child with a walking stick and frame, the latter not so different in principle and construction from the contemporary triangular walking frames. The common modern-day walking (pulpit or zimmer) frame enables people who are unstable to walk, prevents muscle deterioration and prolongs relative independence and autonomous living. Contemporary developments go further. The PAMAID (Personal Adaptive Mobility) robot, for instance, is designed for people who are frail and blind; it 'thinks' for the user through laser and sonar sensors that operate in three modes: a 'manual' mode which functions as a conventional walking frame but emits audible warnings of static and moving obstacles, left and right turns, t-junctions and door openings; an 'aggressive' mode which controls the steering and navigates around obstacles; and a 'shared control' mode to reduce the risk of collision by making adjustments to the user's path. A device combining a mechanical orthosis and electrodes enhances the motor function of paretic wrist muscles in tetraplegic patients, providing greater mobility and independence to people previously highly dependent on others. The dividing line between those able to take advantage of such technology and those who cannot is one of access to resources. Sophisticated robotic equipment is not standard government issue, and is beyond the reach of most people who might find such technology liberating.

Plastic and reconstructive surgeries are part of a suite of procedures and technologies used to redress the disadvantages of difference. Like other kinds of surgeries and body modifications, these have a long history. Medical contracts dating from the sixteenth century were already documenting corrective surgery, such as for inguinal hernia and defective palate, but resection and reconstructive surgery increased significantly with developments in anesthesia and asepsis in the 1800s. Thereafter, increasingly sophisticated procedures were introduced in dermatological and skeletal surgery for people with congenital anomalies, tumors, burns or traumatic injury.

Increasingly, too, a range of assistive technologies have developed to assist with the processes of reconstruction and enhancement. Since the late 1980s, robots and navigators with names that allude to their power – da Vinci, Zeus and Puma – have been used in surgery and to produce medical equipment, prosthetics and hospital beds. Robots are claimed to enhance quality and speed, provide precision control of instruments and enable telesurgery, surgical monitoring and solo performance; in these contexts the robot becomes the 'master slave' of the surgeon (iRobotics 2003). Computer-aided surgery and telemanipulation systems have enhanced surgeons' accuracy, dexterity and visualization with particular impact on microsurgery on the knee, hip, prostate, uterus, intestine, esophagus, gallbladder, spleen, kidney, thorax, heart, lung and brain. Clinical photography, plastic surgery simulators and plastic manikins that grumble and vomit blood have most recently facilitated professional training. Increasingly, people undergo common but sometimes highly complicated surgical procedures with these technical aids, and the capacity for such innovation and refinements appears to be endless. The flow-on to individuals of developments in science and technology, through research and its translation and adaptation, is a simple corollary of parallel processes in other aspects of everyday life. New products for bodily comfort take advantage of materials from space technology. Pillows made from high density viscoelastic, temperature-sensitive 'memory cells' are promoted as superior because of their technological history, for example, as a side product of "certified space technology from the NASA Space Program," a "breakthrough in sleep technology" (Tempur-Pedic 2002). The lexical combination of technology ('viscoelastic') and anthropomorphism (a pillow with 'memory cells') is a marketing strategy that builds on the various links of the body and society.

As I have suggested in linking contemporary equipment and procedures to their historic prototypes, the technologies of rehabilitation and reconstruction are not static or isolated; they reflect developments in other technical and social fields. The use of computer simulation for decision-making in oral or facial surgery, voice recognition and voice synthesizer equipment to allow speech-to-text and text-to-speech translation, the reattachment of limbs, and now the reconstruction of faces are realities not science fiction. At each moment, technology is harnessed to maximize use and minimize risk.

Marketing the Body

With developments in technique, the success of full face transplants in France in February and China in April 2006, and the additional numbers since then, was a predictable therapeutic development. Microsurgery procedures now allow the transplantation of new skin, bones, noses, chins, lips and ears for people who have lost facial features as a result of cancer, burns, bites and accident. While the usual procedure would be a superficial transplant and retention of the underlying bone structures (hence retaining appearance, to a degree), it is now feasible to transplant bone (Anonymous 2002; Greenwald 2007), and as rehearsed in the popular film *Face/Off* (Woo 1997), a person wishing to assume a new identity can now literally take on a new face and identity. So more pedestrian procedures are depicted and promoted routinely. Weekly magazines sold in supermarkets and news agencies include before-and-after photographs of celebrities who have had cosmetic surgery altering face and body shape, many young and with no bodily anomalies that might even suggest the advantages of such procedures.

Functional body technologies can be readily rationalized in contemporary society on the grounds of both economics and human rights. But other technological interventions have little to do with restitution and rehabilitation. Their introduction is driven far more by consumer economics, whereby contemporary notions of the isomorphism of fitness and beauty, desirability and personal worth, and ideas of choice and mastery over the physical body, converge. The body is a commodity. The company E-sthetics, for example, advertising on the web, uses language that normalizes both negative constructions of body change and the surgical resolution of perceived problems. Of facelifts, the advertising text reads, "Few of us like the signs of aging in our body. The facial skin is the only area we can see these changes on a daily basis. It is not surprising that methods to correct aging change, such as facelifts and blepharoplasty, are some of the most popular operations in cosmetic and plastic surgery" (http://www.e-sthetics.com, July 7, 2009). Advocating plastic surgery after pregnancy, the company observes that "most women enjoy being pregnant and are happy to become mothers. But for some, the physical changes caused by pregnancy can take away some of the joy. If you feel this way, you're not alone." Body sculpture "treats the results of aging obesity, weight loss or increase and the effects of pregnancy." The increasing number of men turning also to plastic surgery reflects "a growth in decision making by men in health care issues," but this is also represented as a civil rights and identity issue, as when offering cosmetic foreskin reconstruction to men circumcised as infants (Hudson 2003).[1] In the Australian suburban press, the promises are spectacular and appeal to a hedonism that presents body parts as accessories. Advertisements for cosmetic surgery clinics offer potential clients the chance to "Reshape your body to suit your spirit. Walk-in, walk-out procedures." On-line advertisements enable potential clients to click onto a problem area, read detailed descriptions of the philosophy of the clinics, the staff, the counseling and consultation procedures, learn about the surgery, recovery and longer term outcomes, and read testimonies from people who have had such procedures and now look and feel younger and enjoy enhanced self-esteem and self confidence. Undergoing cosmetic surgery can now be, legitimately, for entirely superficial reasons: "Maybe it is a problem you have always wanted to fix, maybe a little reward or perhaps it's just about getting more from life. Either way it's all about you" (http://www.ashleycentre.com.au, January 19, 2011).

In recent years, online information has provided increasing technical and personal detail about processes and outcomes, in the interests of informed consent and presumably to head off potential litigation; this is not, of course, a characteristic of small newspaper advertisements which make simpler claims of effective, inexpensive and time-efficient procedures. One clinic, part of an international franchise, advertises a "unique weight loss program without appetite suppressants, miracle shakes or pills," with the promise to readers that *nothing tastes as good as thin feels* (http://www.sureslim.com.au, April 9, 2007). The motto is not unique to SureSlim claims; it is repeated as the lead motto on various web-based advertisements for slimming products. Moreover, governments, science and economics have increasingly joined forces to promote surgery over other measures, including lifestyle changes. The report on obesity in Australia, tabled by the House of Representatives Standing Committee on Health and Ageing in the federal parliament in June 2009, for example, promotes bariatric surgery (in contrast with diet and exercise) as the "most effective way of reducing weight and maintaining weight loss in severely obese patients," arguing that while this should be a measure of last resort, resultant weight loss would reduce risk factors for major illnesses and so the costs associated with their management (Australia 2009:55–58).

As suggested by various writers, the body is experienced as a reflection of the self; body image captures how people perceive themselves and how they think others see them. Scheibe (2000) argues that personal history and identity are integrated with bodily features in individual self-construction, but also that visual affirmation is central to identity. He maintains that people affirm their identity by looking at their reflection:

> When we look into the mirror we do not see an accident. We see and feel an essence. We own our names and our faces, our families, and even our place in the world... as essential elements of our being. These are the starting points for the dramas we enact in the world, and we are careful and selective about how we are transformed by circumstances. We have a general reluctance to change our essential features or to suffer mistakes in how we are called, recognized, acknowledged. (16)

But these ideas of self- and social identity, and the confirmation of the two through reflection, ignore the discordance that takes place for many people in their perception of themselves: the discrepancy between character and physical appearance. In this respect, Goffman's understanding of the self, and the significance of appearance to character, and of body to personhood, provides far better insight into the motivations of men and women for cosmetic surgery and other bodily investments. Goffman (1963) maintains that we objectify our bodies, perceiving them as if looking into a mirror, with the reflection framed in terms of society's views and prejudices. Hence the disquiet when contradictions are exposed in (desired or perceived) social identity and self-identity. Given this, Connie Panzarino (1994) was not merely ironic in entitling her book *The Me in the Mirror*. Mirrors are typically aligned to the height of a person standing, and hence Panzarino (and others in wheelchairs) have a different angle to their physical image. But also, self-image and societal norms interact, one implicating the other in ways that shape societal accommodation of the individual. There is disjunction then between the body in the mirror, the body that others might see and the self within the body. Women's and, to a lesser extent, men's anxieties regarding their bodies reflect their understanding of how life choices are shaped by the ways that society 'reads' character and worthiness from physical appearance, and abnegates capability in those who divert from cultural norms. This contributes to the decisions people make regarding body modification and behavior, superficial and extensive, mundane and extreme, including in relation to dress style, adornment, exercise and diet. Prosthetics, cosmetics and surgery are technologies that allow people to manipulate, disguise or correct body structure and function that impede social engagement, interaction and life course.

Men and women with physical disabilities experience disjuncture between who they feel they are and how others see them. Irving Zola looks in the mirror at himself "fully naked for perhaps the first time in twenty years," and is struck by the reality of his own morphology and the power of normative notions of the body and physical and intellectual abilities: "The adjective 'wasted' stuck in my throat. Overdeveloped from the waist up, underdeveloped from the waist down" (Zola 1982:217). Commenting on his disproportionate musculature, Zola continues, "No wonder so many people worried how far this 'below-the-waist' underdevelopment went" (217–218).

Women's identity is still structured persistently by the norms of conventional femininity, leading many to make decisions to alter their bodies to conform to contemporary notions of feminine beauty and the promise of confidence, happiness, fulfillment, success and security. This is not to suggest that women are passively complicit with an ideology that prejudges them – as successful businesswomen or marriage partners – on the basis of their appearance; thirty-five years of feminist activism and wide social and cultural change have at least shaken these presumptions. Kathy Davis (1995), instead, has maintained that women are active in exercising power in this context, when deciding to have cosmetic surgery, so taking as 'reasonable' steps to address 'the problem of ordinariness' and the difficulties they have in negotiating the self with 'bodily deficiencies.' Cosmetic surgery, she argues, has the potential to improve women's self-image and so, for those who are profoundly self-conscious of and inhibited by what they perceive to be embodied inadequacy, enhancing their ability to interact with others. Davis offers the example of a woman who, until she had facial surgery for marked irregularities, always saw herself "as if … in a mirror, seeing herself through the eyes of others" (81). Cosmetic surgery therefore reduces socially isolating physical anomalies or normalizes 'deviant' bodies, so enabling women and men to escape their subjugation to their bodies, to minimize or dissolve through technical means the bodily anomalies that marginalize and disable them (179–181). But these arguments do nothing to challenge a society that includes and rewards people on the basis of the conformity of their appearance, fails to tackle the relationship, and discrepancies, between normative and socially valued appearance, and sidesteps clients' own complicity in maintaining this hegemony.

Women especially incorporate in their self-perception the gaze of others, assessing and maintaining self-awareness of their physical appearance through such refraction, such that, in Leder's terms, they are not "full co-subjectivities, free to experience from a tacit body" (1990:99). But it can be more extreme than this: the promotion of bodily norms, reflected in product advertisements, film and video, skews individuals' perceptions and identity, and shapes obsession in disturbing ways. This is a theme pursued by Hiroshi Teshigahara in his film *The Face of Another* (1966) (see chapter 3). In her book *Autobiography of a Face*, Lucy Grealy (1994) again provides an especially powerful illustration of the alienation that can occur with facial irregularity. She writes of the "singularity of meaning" of her face and its distortion following surgery for Ewing's sarcoma:

> I was my face, I was ugliness – though sometimes unbearable, [it] also offered a possible point of escape. It became the launching pad from which to lift off, the one immediately recognizable place to point when asked what was wrong with my life. Everything led to it, everything receded from it – my face as a personal vanishing point. (7)

Grealy writes of the enormous personal pain and isolation as a result of living with what she saw as a mutilated face, leading her to have had, at the time that she wrote the autobiography, over thirty operations:

> I knew to expect a scar, but how had my face sunk in like that? I didn't understand. Was it possible I'd looked this way for a while and was only just noticing it, or was this change very recent? More than the ugliness I felt, I was suddenly appalled at the notion that I'd been walking around unaware of something that was apparent to everyone else. A profound sense of shame consumed me. (111–112)

Grealy's image ate up her sense of worth. Her looking-glass image was so shocking that she avoided her reflection, such that "the journey back to my face was a long one ... to own the face as my own" (220). It was never a permanent journey: she continued to have surgery, and then, devastated by the unremitting failure of surgeons to restore her jaw and allow her to talk, eat, kiss and laugh with ordinary ease, she turned to the prescription drug OxyContin, then heroin; she died of an apparent overdose in 2002. But in *Autobiography of a Face*, the most poignant aspects of her life are largely unwritten: her twin sister Sarah, non-identical yet no less her living mirror, her Dorian Gray, is mentioned only once.

While surgery might, following Davis, be seen as a legitimate response to marked disfigurement where beauty, femininity and social worth are aligned, it is far more often an instance of women's vulnerability to and acceptance of dominant cultural notions of the feminine, when women opt for breast surgery, for example, because they feel not 'real' women if they have small breasts, or feel objectified if well-endowed. Again, easy access to surgery has shifted body practice. Increasingly, among women from diverse backgrounds in both highly industrialized and poor countries, the ordinary tricks of body disguise – padded bras, tissue paper and handkerchiefs, cleverly cut clothing – are displaced by new, surgically-created breasts, promoted in surprising ways. Radio stations over the past several years have offered breast enlargement as a competition prize, attracting statements of condemnation from some cosmetic surgeons but little other action (National Organization for Women 2004; Cabron 2006). American Broadcasting Company's television program *Extreme Makeover*, broadcast in twenty countries including in Europe and Asia, and in Australia, further highlights how changes to bodily appearance are coupled with the promise of happiness.

Artists have taken the front line in challenging the illusion that cosmetic surgery can ever be the exercise of agency alone. French artist Orlan most notably has played with cultural and historic notions of the body and representation through performance and what she calls 'carnal art,' as the potential transgressions of esthetic surgery began to take hold. From 1990 to 1993, she made a series of filmed and live-broadcast surgical performances in which she transformed the surgical theatre and her own body into the site of performance (www.orlan.net, January 19, 2011). Among her most recent work are digitally-manipulated photo-works that allow greater dynamism and exploration of possible, alternative self-representations.[2]

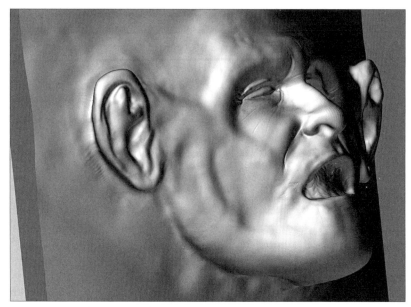

Figure 2.5 Stelarc, *Partial Head*. Heide Museum of Modern Art, Melbourne; 2006. Image by Vincent Wan. Courtesy of Stelarc.

By transforming her features to converge with conventional yet varied notions of beauty, Orlan's 'carnal art' challenges the social and surgical construction of beauty, but also provides an ethical standpoint from which to measure developments in medicine and biology. The framing of her work as art, and her explicit statements of purpose, protect Orlan from the disapprobation directed to others who have had serial cosmetic surgery. In contrast, for example, Jocelynne Wildenstein, the 'cat woman,' has typically been held up as an example of personal folly and female vulnerability as she subjected to the knife, wielded by her surgeon husband, to maintain culturally acceptable good looks. Cindy Jackson is the 'Barbie Doll woman' who from 1988 over a period of sixteen years underwent nine cosmetic surgeries which provide a compendium of esthetic operations. As described on her web-page and in her autobiography, *Living Doll* (Jackson 2002), these included upper and lower eye lid surgery; two rhinoplasties; chin reconstruction; cheek implantation; chemical face peels; face lifts; a fat transfer into her face, lips, nose and mouth lines (her 'smile') from her buttocks; dermabrasion on most of her face; teeth caps, liposuction on her stomach, thighs (twice) and knees; breast implants and a buttock lift;

hair transplants, and permanent makeup tattoos. In her efforts to meta-
morphose into a living doll, the disproportionate and improbable Barbie
in search of a human Ken – a possibility with Steve Erhardt's similar pursuit of fantasy surgery (http://independentsources.com/2005/ 08/21/
butt-implants) – Jackson is a real life example of Fay Weldon's *The Life and
Loves of a She-Devil* (1983).

Celluloid Cyborgs

The cultural production of imagined relations between bodies and
mechanics that emerged throughout the twentieth century fed the imagination of the cyborg, and anticipated and fuelled contemporary anxieties
about the practicalities, ethics and morality of technological incursions.
Technological developments, including refinements in microsurgery and
the use of robots in medicine, while promoted typically because of their
effectiveness, efficiency and successful long-term outcomes, are consistently coupled with nervousness about the deployment of technology to
'normalize' and homogenize people. Fears of the uncontrolled pursuit of
embodied perfection, and fears of displacing human labor with machines,
both have a long history, paralleling and sometimes anticipating the developments of the technologies themselves. These themes were captured
vividly in nineteenth century gothic fiction and older fairly tales, and have
been revisited regularly in the twentieth and early twenty-first century
in contemporary horror and science fiction novels, short stories, mass
popular cultural writing and commercial film. Some of this work, including classic novels such as *Brave New World* (Huxley 1983 [1932]), *Animal
Farm* (Orwell 1945) and *Nineteen Eighty-Four* (Orwell 1949) and the film
The Invasion of the Body Snatchers (Siegel 1956) are allegories of political
and economic formations rather than (simply) portents of medically-
and technically-engineered dystopias, but the allegories work, of course,
because the fear of dystopia is already in place. The larger genre of creative
fantasy and pulp fiction, commercial cinema and art-house film, comics
and cartoons, includes a common fascination with metamorphosis, xenog-
raphy, the android or cyborg, and the potentials of biotechnology, with
story lines that tease the imagination, push the boundaries of present-day
science, and use fantasy and horror to explore contemporary and rehearse
future moral dilemmas. Twentieth century writers such as Dick (1968),
Russ (1985 [1975]), Piercy (1976) and Gibson (1984), for instance, all
played with alternatives of biology, reproduction and interdependence

with technology that are no longer particularly fanciful in the twenty-first century, when the first 'test-tube babies' are adults and assisted reproductive technology and surrogacy are commonplace.

The relationship of humans and machines was explored filmically perhaps first in 1926 in *Metropolis* (Lang 1926), reflecting much earlier worries about industrialization, and the resistance of workers to mechanization and fears of redundancy, should machines prove both cheaper and more efficient. Other early films simply portray humans as stripped of humanity to become as if robots under changing conditions of production, and illustrate debates within politics, dating from the nineteenth century, regarding the alienation of workers. Charlie Chaplin's factory worker in *Modern Times*, and the film's depiction of the mechanization of everyday life, drew on debates during the Great Depression (see Wood 2002:60). Chaplin was prophetic about the costs of routine, anticipating that the machinery itself, the specificity of tasks and the pace of the work, would destroy bodies and alienate labor – he presaged repetitive strain injury and a range of other occupational health problems.

These themes have been revisited constantly in films and television serials that include humanoid robots and robot-controlled humans.

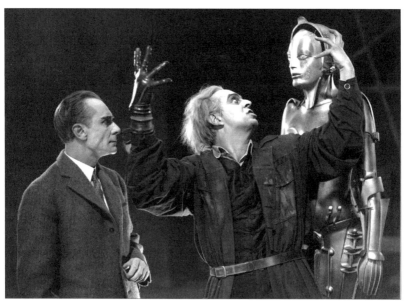

Figure 2.6 *Metropolis,* Germany, director Fritz Lang; 1927.
Courtesy of Photofest.

Consider the women in *The Stepford Wives* (1975, 2004), *Star Trek's* Data *(1966–)*, the replicants in *Blade Runner* (1982); humans transformed into robots *Robocop* (1987); humans endowed with robot qualities and super strength in various films of *Superman* (1978–), and television series such as the *Six Million Dollar Man* (1974–1978) and *Bionic Woman* (1976–1977); about humans who appear normal but become mental robots; and of aliens that replicate humans – *Total Recall* (1990), *Invasion of the Body Snatchers* (1956, 1978), *A Clockwork Orange* (1971).

Lindsay Anderson's films particularly resonate with these themes and this book. *If* (1968) was the first of a trilogy of films about anomie and structural chaos, introducing the central character, Mick Travis (played by Malcolm McDowell). In the second of the films, *O Lucky Man* (1973), Travis, now a coffee salesman, leases his body to Professor Millar (Graham Crowden), and flees the research hospital after witnessing an outcome of Millar's research – in a scene that repulsed me more than most over the years – a human head grafted onto a convulsing hippopotamus-like body. The entire action at the Millar Research Clinic is ten minutes of a 186-minute film; the scene in question lasts less than one minute. Travis enters the research hospital after escaping from torture and near death at a military installation. He volunteers to participate in the research program, and after a series of tests, Millar informs him:

> Michael, I don't know if anyone's ever told you this, but you happen to belong to a very rare group of encephaloids.

> *What's that supposed to mean?*

> Essentially, it means you are in a position to be particularly helpful to us in our research.

> *What kind of research?*

> What do you think are the most successful animals that have ever lived in this world?

> *The ants.*

> The dinosaur.

Millar continues:

> Mankind has only one hope – science. Technology is the survival kit of the human race. Even the politicians realize this…. The technical solutions are already within our power … it's only a matter of

learning to live in a new way.... With present transplant techniques, there is no reason why everyone shouldn't live to be 250 or 300 years old instead of our present miserable 70 or 80 years. We are on the verge of a whole series of discoveries that will transform our conceptions of human life.

What's all this got to do with me?

Michael, at this very moment, in laboratories throughout the world, life is being created. It's only a matter of years, perhaps even months, before we can begin to produce a whole generation of new and far more fully adapted creatures ... computers, DNA molecules ... This is the future. This is the work for which I need your help.

Yes, but what's going to happen to me? Will I come out the same as I went in?

Not the same. Better.

Mick Travis bargains the amount of money he will receive for the lease of his body, and he is put into a bed in a private room – he becomes a patient. Concerned about what will now happen to him, he sneaks into another room and discovers what appears to be a young man of around his own age, shaking, terrified, aphasic – his head has been grafted onto a convulsing animal body. Travis screams in horror, jumps out of a window and escapes.

In the final film of this trilogy, *Britannia Hospital* (1982), Travis and Millar meet again. The specific storylines of this genre are repeated, shifting from pure fantasy to near future. Travis is an investigative reporter. Millar is now a highly successful experimental scientist whose opus magnum is to be a patchwork human made from cryopreserved body parts. Travis discovers the refrigeration room, and through misadventure, causes the head intended for the constructed human to defrost. Travis pays the ultimate price: he is beheaded so that his head can be used on the compositional body. The experiment is a disaster. Travis's head tears away from the body; the body remains murderous until destroyed. With the failure of this experimental man-made man, an alternative experimental achievement is unveiled to an audience that includes the Queen Mother and her acolytes (played by actors in ways that furthered notions of bodily transgression). The achievement is Genesis, a living cerebellum linked to artificial intelligence, a new human being of pure brain, devoid of what Millar calls the 'effectual' body. The film was not a success, apparently because viewers failed to appreciate its satire and instead simply saw it as "excessive and off-key" (Holm 2002).

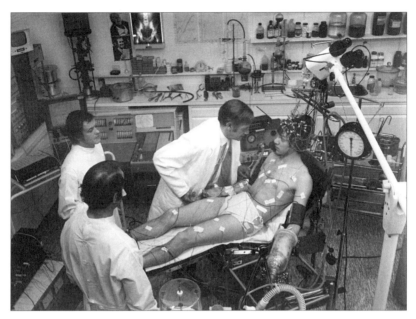

Figure 2.7 *O Lucky Man,* UK, director Lindsay Anderson; 1973.
Courtesy of Photofest.

The idea of a monstrous human composed from distinct cadaverous body parts, depicted in *O Lucky Man* and *Brittania Hospital*, dates from Shelley's *Frankenstein* (1818) and its various filmic incarnations and variants.[3] The theme reappears in an episode of the original *Taggart* series on Scottish Television (STV) (1983), in which a serial killer seeks to make a body for himself. In the film *Mr. Stitch* (1996), Lazarus, created out of body parts from eighty-eight different donors, is tormented by visions or memories of his donors. An extraordinary number of films on grafting and personality transfer exist. These include *The Incredible 2-Headed Transplant* (1971) and *The Mind Snatchers* (1972) (also released as *The Happiness Cage* and *The Demon Within*), both of which treat the head, mind and personality as identical and pursue the theme of embodied memory. These films largely derive from or appear to be inspired by Maurice Renard's novel *Les Mains d'Orlac* (*The Hand of Orlac*), which Thorpe (1998) in turn links to the Grimm Brothers' story, *The Tale of the Three Army Surgeons* (see also Goldberg 2002). The first film with this motif appears to be Edison's film *The Thieving Hand* (1908), in which a passer-by purchases a prosthetic arm for an armless beggar. The arm has memories of its own, and continues its life of theft until reunited with its rightful owner in prison. Landsberg (1995:239) suggests that "through the prosthetic arm, the beggar's body manifests memories of actions that it, or he, never actually committed. In fact, his memories are radically divorced from lived experience and yet they motivate his actions.... The film underscores the way in which memory is constitutive of identity." Remakes and variations followed, including Oliver Stone's *The Hand* (1991), based on Marc Brandel's novel *The Lizard's Tail* of a cartoonist who loses his drawing hand in an accident and who becomes obsessed that his lost hand is stalking his enemies. In *Body Parts* (1991), the arm of a killer is grafted onto the arm of a crime psychologist, with violent results; in *The Amazing Transplant* (1970), the anatomy with a life of its own is a penis. And, in an extension of relationship of self to part, in *The Fifth Element* (1997), scientists recreate a woman, destroyed in a space explosion, from the DNA in the remains of her hand. In this scenario, the woman is her hand, and the hand is the sum of the parts. Brian Jacobs (1999), who claims that over

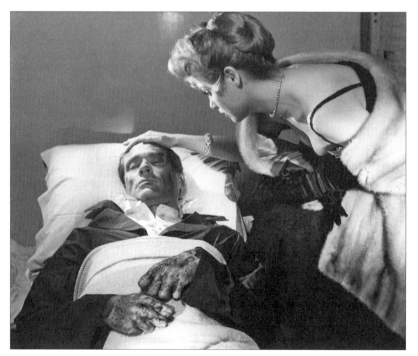

Figure 2.8 *The Hands of Orlac,* U.S., director Edmond T. Gréville; 1960. Courtesy of Photofest.

one hundred films derive from the original Orlac story, suggests that these films reveal a significant characteristic of our cultural imagination; his observation that "body parts associated with a criminal deed are, in our minds, invested with the human spirit behind the deed" (8) was made in response to life-imitating-art, when it was disclosed that Matthew Scott, the world's third hand transplant, was recipient of the hand of a convicted murderer whose suicide had allowed the transplant. The theme has also been transported into advertisements – in Australia, a roving tongue in search of a cold beer.[4]

In her discussion of films of possessed hands, Goldberg (2002; also Feinberg 2001) suggests links between the 'rogue hand' with neurological disorders and psychological/ontological dilemmas of the location of self. Goldberg's reflections are echoed in contemporary debates about transplantation and the underlying concerns of people who are or might be donors or recipients; narratives of transplantation/transformation explore "*how we become monstrous to ourselves*: how the ambiguous self is revealed to be more monstrous than any external horror, and how true horror is rooted in the vulnerability of our physical form. It is a transformation which makes manifest the unreliable nature of both body and mind.... Can the self fracture and yet be restored to integrity?" (3–4, emphasis in original). This suggests an existential dilemma in the relationship between body and soul, corporeality, memory and emotion. Commonly, a physician reassures a patient that following transplantation or other surgery, he or she will be a 'new man' or a 'new woman.' Indeed, that is the fear. The notion of bodily integrity and the possibility of organic (or cellular) memory is a common concern among people who have had transplants and among their partners. In a documentary shown in a prime time television program in Australia, *Reality Bites* (2002), the wife of a man who has just undergone a heart transplant explains her fears: she fell in love with his old heart, not this new one. The surgeon reassures her that "it's only an organ"; the heart does not remember. But the possible transportability of the personal qualities of a donor adds to the anxiety of organ recipients (see chapters 6 and 7).

Given anxiety about provenance, and links between body parts and personality, it is not surprising that films of transplantations and related body experiments are largely constructed as horror or science fiction films, as described above, even when the science is increasingly familiar. The horror derives from the fact that these films "underscore the vulnerability of body parts: the fear of losing a part of your body constitutes a primal source of horror" (Wilson 1995:250). The focus is not on the lived effect of loss, but on the existential consequences of bodily distortions and reconstruction, the nature of the self, and the relationship between the body surface and 'true'/inner self, corporeality and being. The horror in the face of the man who Mick Travis discovers in *O Lucky Man* captures this precisely: he is still sentient, horribly aware that he (his self, located in his transplanted head) is trapped in/attached to a non-human body. Conflicts arise even over changes in substance of the body and definitions of self, as reflected in concerns about blood transfusion not because of fear of infection but because of anxieties about the connections between substance and self, distortions of the self and bodily integrity (Singelenberg 1990).

Scientific, biomedical and biotechnical advances and their ethical implications are reported routinely in the mass media. While science programs and essays conventionally emphasize their incremental developments and values for the common good, the potential breaches in human rights and social justice are also often part of this picture. This is perhaps especially so where ethical issues have not been resolved, or where there is substantial community dissent. As Margaret Lock (2001) so eloquently illustrates, cadaver transplantation is problematic especially where there is disagreement on the timing of death. Again, science fiction and horror films conventionally draw on the archetypal scientist-as-god (or evil incarnate) to pursue the morality tales that underpin resistance to such science. For example, in *Species* (1995), a simple twist on Shelley's Frankenstein, scientists create a murderous creature by combining human and alien DNA. The films frequently also address other contemporary social issues. *Gattaca* (1997), on genetic engineering, could be read as a filmic presage of possibilities and certainly reflects the worries set out in political debates about genetic research, prenatal screening, gamete donation and the threats of modern eugenics. While cloning is controversial in part because of the use of embryonic stem cells in societies where the nature of life and the status of the embryo are in dispute, the debates surrounding experimentation address, too, the fear that technological advances will lead to increased control over reproduction, favoring the perfect and selecting against possible disability (Squier 2004).

Successes in cloning in other species, and the potential transferability of techniques to humans, have been linked increasingly to the demand for spare parts and hence to transplantation surgery, and again, the time frame now of these debates has largely shifted the level of anxiety. Following the successful cloning of the sheep Dolly (after Dolly Parton), *The Age*

(Melbourne) in 1997 introduced an article on the tensions between the technical wherewithal to clone and the ethics of cloning, with the sub-headings "We may one day be flocking after Dolly" and "The replaceable you." Two years later, in the United States, an advanced cloning method, using the nuclei of connective-tissue cells of bovine fetuses (fibroblasts) as the genetic template, resulted in the birth of three healthy, identical calves: a breakthrough in the search for "a system for genetic modification and large-scale cloning in cattle" with a success rate significantly better than that of the Scottish researchers who created Dolly (Cibelli, Stice, Golueke, Kane, Jerry, Blackwell, de Leon, Robl 1998). Cloning is repre-sented commonly now in popular representations as at the cutting edge of medical science, providing efficient and faster ways of making transgenic fetuses for cell therapies and adult animals for protein production and organs for xenotransplantation. It is a field represented as rich with com-mercial potential to develop interventions against disease, a perspective that inevitably feeds into prejudices and anxieties about the megaloma-nia of heroic science, the imagined directions of contemporary clinical research, and the moral, ethical and political dilemmas that such research augurs despite legislative steps, in Australia in 2007, to permit somatic cell nuclear transfer (i.e. therapeutic cloning). It takes little time for the anx-ious hype to mellow; routinely I am asked about stem cell therapy to repair my limp left arm.

Performing Disability

I want to return here to the more modest technical advances with which I began this chapter. The simplest technology extends the body's capacity, even if, in consequence, the body loses its spontaneity and other freedoms. An 'intelligent' walker like the PAMAID robot is only as good as its soft-ware, and presumably it can make errors – confusing a stair step with a ledge, for example. Moreover, even when the technology is integrated into a body – lodged internally or fused, as is the case with a pacemaker – still the body is always a cultural hybrid. At its simplest, clothed, it is already encumbered and elaborated, protected and adorned. At any given time, too, the biological structures of the body are modified through connection to a robotic mechanism or a simple technology (a telephone, a wooden stick): these inventions are now everyday prostheses, technologies to help us live our lives. The role of prostheses and reconstructive surgery is partly (some might argue entirely) a pragmatic response to lack or loss, a means by which rehabilitation is enabled as a physical, psychological and social project. As already argued, such measures disguise or minimize the visual barriers of impairment for the person affected and for others with whom she or he interacts, allowing the person to find harmony for the body in the mirror, the body that others might see, and the self within the body.

Yet not all people are comfortable with prostheses: the technologies themselves, while enabling greater function, underline the departure of the individual from normatively able bodies. Consider Nancy Mairs's sense of shame, as she described her emotion, when she became dependent on a wheelchair for mobility (1987, 1996). Others adopt an agentive approach. Andre Dubus appropriates his wheelchair as a signifier of success, for example, as do many of the men with whom I have worked over the past decade: here are men who are still powerful and active (Miner 1997; Manderson and Peake 2005). Gender and sexuality play a clear role in people's accommodation of disability and their willingness to embrace and exploit bodily difference, as I explore in later chapters.

Many people, in addition, live with conditions that do not allow them to merge into a crowd and appear like 'everyone else,' nor is there the technology to minimize or disguise difference. By way of example, I want to reflect on the text and visual works of Ju Gosling (1997–2005), whose critical approach to disability, her interest in cybertechnology, and her own need for a prosthetic led her to create a persona around disablement that illustrates how identity can be constructed in an alternative mode. I conclude this chapter by discussing her work, as a means of furthering an appreciation of the desire for conformity (and of being 'normal') and the positioning that is involved when someone resists rather than complies.

Gosling is an English artist, trained as a dancer and working with digital lens-based media, performance and text, interactive installations, photography and film. Although she is well known by the name Ju Gosling, her nom-de-net, Ju90, frees her of the constraints of gender, age, race, sexuality and disability, so making explicit the social construction of identity and the ability of people to operate independently of this, in cyberspace at least. In adolescence, Gosling developed Scheuermann's Disease, a condition of the thoracic and lumbar spine caused by a growth abnormality, in which the posterior part of the growth plate, but not the anterior, continues to grow, leading to kyphosis (rounding) and osteochondrosis (ossification). The condition is more common in men than women, a detail that perhaps pleases Gosling, given her own play with gender. In severe cases, it causes continued pain. Gosling describes the affected area of her back as "stiff and inflexible"; she experiences chronic inflammation, pain, tendonitis and muscle spasms. Everyday routine activities exacerbate the pain – sitting, holding the phone, being bumped on the street, traveling on buses, being touched. Gosling was advised to wear a body brace, a standard means to manage both the curvature and discomfort; out of this material item, she forged her identity as a disabled woman. The original orthosis was skin-pink plastic, covering the full length of her spine and fastened with nylon straps. It exaggerated her waist and hips while exposing her breasts, creating what she saw as a feminized, almost Edwardian silhouette. It was impossible to wear her usual clothing with the brace:

> I felt my identity dissolve; the brace had claimed me, borg-like, to wear it. I fitted into the brace, but the brace did not fit me. My androgynous image had vanished; instead the brace/borg exaggerated my femininity and impairment whilst conflating the two…. Trapped within the borg/brace, … the only answer was to reassert my ownership, to assimilate the brace within myself rather than continuing to be assimilated by it. (www.ju90.co.uk/cylife3.htm)

Wilson (1995) has argued that while "a machine both sheds parts and acquires new ones easily … the human perspective seems to insist upon organic integrity as the only possible norm" (246). But this is not an option for people who need technical and mechanical apparatus in order to live. For Gosling, the project was one of the brace itself, working with it as an item of material culture, to reconstitute it and, by so doing, to recreate her own identity from 'borg' to 'cyborg.' The uniform appearance of standard orthotic and prosthetic equipment, particular those that are relatively inexpensive and/or available through government health schemes, depersonalize, reducing individuals to their physical limitations and to the stereotypes that inform them. Even small resistance therefore has an impact: Gosling notes the difference it made to her, and others' reactions to her, of a custom-carved walking-stick which signified "something very different to the standard metal, medical aid – its unique appearance restore(d) its associations with gender-bending, clowning and discipline, as well as, in this case, having connotations of paganism and shamanism – but it performs exactly the same task" (www.ju90.co.uk/cylife4.htm). A personalized aid, Gosling notes, reveals the social identity of the user. Indeed, the item may or may not be prosthetic: who is to know?

In 1996, Gosling worked with costume designer Jo Lang to transform the brace. The goal was not to hide the brace and thereby hide the physical condition that required it, but to step outside of the medical and social spaces of disability. In doing so, Gosling drew on her own cyborg-augmented identity through glasses and contact lenses, Psion palmtop computer and mobile phone, and her sexual and social identity as queer, androgynous and non-nonconformist. She drew, too, on surf and cyberpunk imagery. The brace was sprayed metallic silver and decorated with found objects, mementos and paraphernalia of the technological environment: a shattered CD, placed partially over the area of spinal degeneration, symbolized the obsolescence of technology and the challenge of change; a decorative loop attached to a shell gave her a way to carry items such as keys; the nylon straps were padded and decorated: "My brace now became my friend and my protector, the exterior mark of my interior pain, a removable, tattooed,

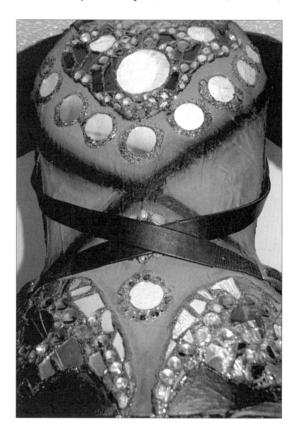

Figure 2.9
Ju Gosling, *Detail of Brace*; 2001.
© Ju Gosling aka Ju90.

exoskeleton, my armour" (www.ju90.co.uk/cylife5.htm). The inflexibility of the brace demanded also a change in style of clothing, for which purpose Gosling drew on the BDSM (bondage-domination/sadist-masochist) referents for the corset-like appearance of the brace and her use of a stick, evoking orthopedic fetishism, the notion of the dominatrix and the transformation of the brace itself into an object of desire. BDSM, she argued, provided a performative, narrative sexuality that explored power, control and trust. Now sleek and black, dancer and camp performance artist, cyborg complete, Ju was ready to perform disAbility.

A few but growing numbers of people other than Gosling have followed this path of performed disability, prepared to make a spectacle of their selves in order to reclaim public space from which they have been excluded as a result of their disability. Raimund Hoghe, a contemporary German dancer with marked scoliosis, uses his naked back as part of his dance performance; Bill Shannon, 'the crutch-master,' incorporates his crutches to support his body in order to perform his own intensely physical dance style.[5] My hand brace plays a similar role, provoking people to ask me directly whether I am wearing an orthotic brace or jewelry; my reply that it is both brace and jewelry typically, intentionally, confuses. There are other examples: the squashed soft drink cans that cover the spine of a prosthetic leg on one young man, depicted in Kath Duncan's film *My One-Legged Dream Lover* (1999), for instance, and the more common examples of people who use prosthetic 'hands' with functional hooks or claws rather than a disguised non-functional hand with fingers, and prosthetic legs worn without covers or with flamboyantly patterned fiberglass protective sheaths.

Physical and psychological factors are central considerations for most, if not all, plastic and reconstructive surgeries. But as suggested above, the esthetic guidelines for surgery are shaped by cultural values of the normal and pathological, beauty and ugliness, and such qualities, in turn, are entangled with moral qualities, happiness and personal success. The social importance of these values, in turn, irrespective of functional capacity, encourages individuals to minimize or to dissolve, through surgery or other technical means, bodily anomalies that they believe to be disabling.

The focus on perfect bodies, on threats to bodily integrity and the symbolism of embodied deviance in films, novels and in the everyday behavior of people, highlights how bodies take on multiple meanings and tones, how posture, gesture, voice and text all bend to cultural orthodoxies and refract from them. Body maintenance, diet and dress, and the contemporary bodily phenomena of anorexia nervosa, cosmetic surgery, and body building involving the misuse of hormones all highlight the work that bodies do in meaning making and as vehicles to other points. Bodily exhibitions and investments, obsessions and neuroses, emphasize the need to understand how individuals with bodily change make adjustments in their self-perception and their relations to others.

The settings of the succeeding chapters in this book are of contemporary industrialized society and medicine. As illustrated above, this context includes somewhat fanciful reflections on science and technology, and on advanced surgical techniques and transplants, developments in immunotherapy, and the emerging possibilities as a result of advances in genetics, microsurgery and pharmacology. Many of these advances are taken for granted, provided that those in need of interventions have the personal resources and access to them. The everyday technologies with which this chapter opened are cases in point. Other developments are regarded with ambivalence: the advantages of particular technologies to the individual countered by fears of their impact more widely, fears fed by images of medicine out-of-hand, excesses of surgery and biological experiment. The result is a see-saw of experimental science and technical know-how, evidenced by the marvel of the double-hand transplant, on the one hand, and the foreboding of human cloning on the other.

In this context, on an everyday basis, people must make decisions, or come to terms with decisions made for or taken from them that involve fundamental changes to bodily functions and appearance. Below, I extend the enquiry into the body and its meanings beyond examples of body decoration and form, and explore the loss of body parts, functions and/ or appearance following illness or accident. I turn to the embellishments, absences, elaborations and demise of the bodies of people who have not, for reasons of their health, enjoyed the agency that is seen to characterize contemporary cultures of the body. My interest is in how they understand the surface changes to their bodies, and bodily disruptions to and below the surface, and how these changes affect how they see themselves. I explore how changes in body image affect people as social beings. I consider how they challenge, resist, redefine and re-establish their own identities through body surface and boundary. These people provide converse cases to the norm; their experiences and viewpoints provide us with a window by which to better understand the nature of embodiment. Contrarily, while cyborg invention, cyber communication and virtual worlds might suggest that the physical body has been superseded, the body has never been so present as a commodity, technology and symbol. Deliberate bodily modification is, at least superficially, evidence of control. But, at a time of unprecedented agency and technical skill available to those with sufficient resources, large numbers of people must negotiate their lives via constraints to their physical bodies, stripped of the usual ways to access and build on social membership and identity. Unwanted and largely unforeseen modifications, loss of function, failure and decline are evidence of the body – both social and physical – out of control. Their challenge is to find ways, beyond or despite their physicality, of asserting authority, claiming authenticity and agency, and so personhood.

Notes

1. URL: http://www.phudson.com/GENITAL/uncircumcision.html, accessed May 4, 2006.

2. See Orlan's home page (http://www.orlan.net) for biographic and bibliographic information; see also various articles in *Body & Society* 5(2–3) (1999) and Clark (2002).

3. See Shelley (1985/1818). Numerous films have been based on the novella; many others deal with hospitals and experimentation: people are turned into automatons controlled by a remote-control device *Horror Hospital* (1973); an insane doctor creates a machine to reanimate his dead wife in *The Dead Hate the Living* (1999); Frankenstein (1958) returns to create a creature from various body parts with the brain of his assistant, hunchbacked dwarf; and the son of Frankenstein (1970) makes a human from dead body parts (Sangster 1970).

4. Toohey's Extra Dry Commercial, see http: //www.youtube.com/watch ?v=4tML1z720C4, 10 September 2007.

5. Shannon's performance was observed in Melbourne in October 2005, see http://www.virtual provocateur.com, website last accessed July 8, 2009; Hoghe performed in the Melbourne International Arts Festival, October 2003; see http://www.raimundhoghe.com, website last accessed July 8, 2009.

3

Visible Ruptures: The Art of Living with Lack

Normality is narratively surprising. (Eco 2000:5–6)

Popular culture and its products, I have demonstrated, anticipate and track developments in science and technology, and in so doing challenge the nature of the normal, the realm of the imaginable, and the transformation of the impossible to the possible. These are not acts of the imagination of the twenty-first century. Origin myths and fables, magic and sorcery, and the miracles of healing told as articles of faith in formal religions and retold in fine art draw on the world as experienced and yet perplexing. Variations in nature that are at a distance from the familiar and predictable are equally puzzling, mutant and deviant. Creative arts have had much fun playing with changes in form and procedure, while resisting science and technology's efforts to erase abnormality. These fantasies are points of inspiration for and a presage of new knowledge and technical innovation, ways of managing the unpredictable, correcting the problematic, and realizing different practices, appearance or structure.

Set against heroic medicine and the most dramatic techniques of body salvage and renewal, many technologies are easily accessed and designed simply to eradicate or minimize difference through modest disguise, even if presented as superior in function to earlier props: a cochlear implant, a breast implant, a prosthetic leg with computer hydraulics or the capacity for fusing with the bone. These prosthetics can be as invasive as the condition, injury or disease that resulted in the loss of function or sense in the first place, for the introduction of a technology requires its user to reconceptualize bodily functions, capacities and possibilities. In everyday life, without dramatic bodily change, people move in and out of awareness of the body, adapting posture, changing gesture, responding to transient dysfunctions such as a burp, an itch or a mild ache. Leder (1990) maintains

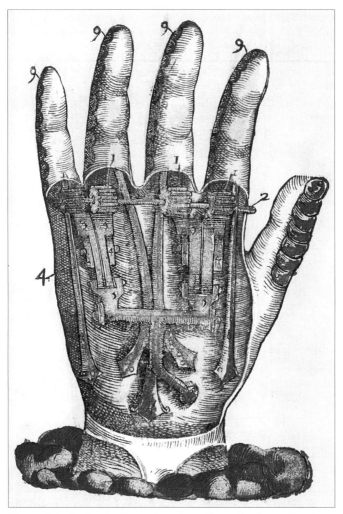

Figure 3.1 Ambroise Pare, drawing of prosthetic mechanical hand; 1564. Courtesy of Wellcome Library, London.

that bodily awareness or presence occurs only when dysfunction interferes with ordinary deportment and habitus. Pain, for instance, inhibits function and motion; profound changes to appearance or function shape how a person sees himself or herself and how he or she interacts with others. In this context, the pathological is constituted as "the disturbance of the normal mechanism ... a quantitative variation, an exaggeration, or attenuation" (Canguilhem 1991:118–119).

Despite developments in microsurgery and the effective use of antibiotics, amputation is often still the only way to deal with severe trauma, prevent necrosis and avoid death. The usual outcome for men and women who lose limbs, depending on their general fitness, mental and physical health, and level of excision, is to be fitted with a prosthesis. With a prosthetic arm or leg, a person gains mobility or dexterity and, in consequence, is able to regain a measure of personal independence. Depending on age, luck and personal resources, he or she may also be able to resume work and other aspects of his or her prior life. For most people, this return to normalcy – based not on body morphology but on social action and engagement – is critical to their wellbeing (Manderson 2005). It is a point captured in a memorable Dali-esque scene in the film *Kandahar* (Makhmalbaf 2001), when Afghani men and women swing on crutches over sand dunes in a race for a parachute drop of artificial legs. In low-income countries, prostheses are difficult to come by, and those of high quality, light and durable, of the sort routinely available in highly industrialized settings, are unattainable. Yet without a simple prosthetic device, everyday life can be unspeakably difficult, creating dependency and leading to deprivation and early death. Those who do not lose limbs, but lose the use of them through stroke or spinal cord injury, have even fewer options without financial resources or adequate state assistance.

While medical practitioners are called on to address immediate changes in the body and signs of pathology, to reduce debility and pain and prevent death, other health professionals are more interested in the continuing tasks of people in rehabilitation and adaptation. People must learn again to use their bodies, resume interrupted activities and/or take up other activities deemed equivalent. In so doing, they seek to re-establish normality in their own terms, on the basis of their past experience, so symbolizing recovery and restitution. Through the physical and social acts of recuperation and rehabilitation, people transit from sickness and incapacitation back to a state of health congruent with particular social and cultural values and conventions of context. "The essential thing is *to have had a narrow escape"* and then return to a normal way of doing and being, "a state in which one notices the body as little as possible outside of the joyous sense of existence" (Canguilhem 1991:119, 122, quoting Jaspers 1913:6). Return from sickness to normality occurs through social action and interaction, not through the fading of pathology or the repair of tissue alone. For those who experience major bodily change, the rehabilitation team is critical. Physicians, therapists, prosthetists and others have the mandate to assist their patients to re-establish a normal life, or to support their adaptation so that they can live a life as normal as possible. While Canguilhem maintains that the healthy individual is one who "measures his health in terms of his capacity to overcome organic crises in order to establish a new order" (1991:200), in effect rehabilitation is about recovering the old order and reclaiming or maintaining a life that is contiguous with life pre-trauma (Warren and Manderson 2008).

In rehabilitation, patients are encouraged to pick up their lives as they were before the interruption with injury or illness, or, with longstanding illness or deterioration, as they might have been. This task can be daunting in the imagination and literally. The body must learn a new language. Individual identity or sense of self is grounded in action, not only in relation to specific activities, interactions and occupation, but also to changes in habitus and social practice; people must first reconcile to the disruptions that have occurred in these fields. With amputation, or with the loss of the function of a limb or limbs as occurs with stroke or neuropathy, the discrepancies between surface and self are stark. What is it like suddenly to lose a limb or to lose the ability to move it, and to discover, later, that the body has now made its own history? How is it – as a result of a vehicle or work accident, a misplaced step, a minor infection that failed to heal, a hidden tumor, or a loss of consciousness barely recalled – that the body's surface can change so quickly and irrevocably? And after the self-centered excitement of the hospital and day visits for rehabilitation, once the basic techniques of prostheses and aids are learned, how do people reclaim and reshape their lives with a body or bodily parts that are often read as a signal of presumed essential change?

Rehabituation

Following loss of function and mobility through injury or disease, a person needs to establish a new sense of embodiment, cognitively, neurologically and physically reorganizing the body schema, re-learning tasks that were near automatic. He or she needs to learn to move without self-consciousness of changes in function and loss. I refer to these tasks as rehabituation – embodied learning involving the recovery or recreation of habitus. I refer therefore to the establishment of habituation – that is, the restoration of old and/or the invention and internalization of new ways of being. Both psychological and physical mechanisms are invoked as, despite fundamental morphological changes, a person gains a renewed

sense of familiarity with his or her body. Post-surgery or following hospitalization, people need to learn to care for the sites of trauma and inability
while reinventing ways of doing. They learn to incorporate their new body
into their body schema, imperfectly and at least superficially, in the everyday practices of bodily response and management. The task of becoming
accustomed to a new/different body is complex, yet once achieved, is
remarkable because of its facility; the body's new limits are incorporated
as habitus, that is, at the level of the subconscious.

The processes of rehabituation and revised habitus are distinct from
rehabilitation, the institutional means and formal process by which
some of this is learned. Rehabilitation emphasizes restorative tasks; it
takes account of the possibility of limits to the restitution of functions
and the reclamation of roles and capabilities. But the task is more than
this, both during the formal process of rehabilitation and subsequently.
Rehabituation involves learning to use the new, changed body without
self-consciousness. Physical and cognitive dimensions to rehabilitation, such as exercise regimes, learning the lexicon and the activities
associated with embodied change, modifications to domestic space, and
equipment, all provide people with the technologies for rehabituation,
but they are not the same as the intuitive incorporation and semi-auto-
matic ways in which the body is used. Posture and gesture, deportment
and motion, action and reaction occur with as little awareness as that of
the healthy body itself; the body is experienced tacitly and is therefore
not a "thematic object of experience" (Leder 1991:1).

Losing mobility, independence and autonomy, fully or partially, strikes
at the heart of cultural understandings of adulthood, and people work hard
to make sense of events of loss. Through formal rehabilitation, as people
gain practical skills to return to work and their everyday lives, they seek
to appropriate and invert ruptures and tragedies so that events instantiate
strength of character and other cultural values: not so much heroism and
determination, though these are present, but will, humility, optimism and
grace. These are not values about which people speak on an everyday basis.

As a first step, in formal rehabilitation, people with amputations are
taught to dress the wound and handle the stump, replace bandages and
socks, prevent pressure sores and manage infections. Depending on the
location of the amputation, suitability of the site and personal readiness,
they may learn to don and doff a prosthesis and begin to use it as a functional appurtenance, to gain or regain muscle strength to transfer their
bodies from bed to wheelchair, and so on. By the time a person has learned

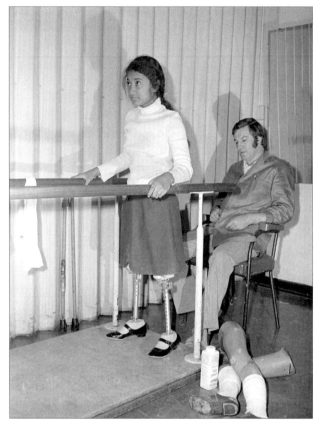

Figure 3.2 Health worker supervises a young girl trying
out a pair of prosthetic legs; 1976. Photograph by Laurie
Richards. Courtesy of Museum Victoria.

to stand and take his or her first steps with a prosthetic leg, then, or turn a
tap with a prosthetic hand, he or she is well on the way to returning home:

> I had accepted it (amputation of both legs) before I even came home
> from hospital. I feel I've been punished in a way because I couldn't
> bear to look at a stump. Now I've got to handle them. And that taught
> me a lesson. And I think it is, they don't look very nice with the scar
> and everything. Still, there are (people) a lot worse off than what I am.
> At least I've got the top of my body. (Jean)

Over time, the atypical pace and routine structure of the hospital become frustrating, and men and women speak of how their

determination to get out of the hospital motivated their commitment to therapy. In demonstrating their ability to care for their bodies, they consequently distanced themselves from the body part that they must now handle. Caring for the body became a skill, the wound and the stump objects of care. Helen recalled:

> Well, your surroundings change completely. You're not where you think you are; you think you're someplace else. I can't remember that I was worried about my leg at the time. Of course I fought so hard to get out. Never missed a physio(therapy) session, although I was doing it all by myself actually. I'd done more than I should have to help myself. I was determined to be back out there as soon as I could. Doing everything they told me to do and trying to do more to help myself. [I wanted to know] how soon can I get another leg on? How long is this going to take to heal up to get this artificial limb so I can get out of here? You feel so useless lying there and needing help for everything. I'd sooner go without than ask anybody for help. But I mean, you can't do that when you're in the position I was in, you've got to have help. But I'd try to do more than I should or do it for myself. It was more important to me to be able to do things on my own. The physiotherapist was astounded with what I could do. I used to do my own bandaging and all of that.

People objectify the body part requiring particular attention in order to manage distress and aversion, for example, in handling the stumps of flesh, and in doing so, they reconstruct their idea of self. It is not the self that has been excised, but the other – *a thing, an object,* even, some people described it, *a child.* Men and women spoke of their grief for their lost limb(s). Amputation was, for those whose surgery was due to disease, a way to prevent imminent death, but in making sense of it, people also began to engage with the inevitable end. Fantasies of the limb restored was a means, one person claimed, of "coming to grips with my mortality, and convincing myself that I am still alive and I am going to live." One woman said that losing a limb was like losing a child, because you're losing part of yourself; one man spoke of losing an old friend; another of being a "murderess" to agree to her foot being amputated. This was a strategy that allowed for disassociation, as the person learned to deal with his or her new body in a way that kept the self intact: *I am normal, it is just that I have one leg.*

Rehabituation takes far longer than the time spent as an inpatient and the transitional period set aside for rehabilitation. But from the beginning of hospitalization, people explore changes in the limits of function, and adjust and incorporate alternative ways of doing, using and reading the body in new ways, from managing edema in a stump to brushing one's hair or answering the phone with the other (or the remaining) hand. Rehabilitation introduces new actions and activities to the person with body loss; over time, these are undertaken increasingly without self-consciousness. Habituation occurs when at least some of these tasks are nearly automatic. This is effected through practice. The 'good' hand reaches for the phone at the first ring tone without the active remembering of the need to do so. The cues to body use, movement and response are internalized; a prosthetic is incorporated into a new 'sensorimotor schema' such that the body boundaries, proprioception and kinesthesia are reconfigured. The process is a continuing one, of evolving mindfulness of the body, its limitations and possibilities.

This mindfulness extends to the practical management of the body to avoid wounds and infection, attend to and manage pressure sores and lesions. Bono, for example, found that local swelling of her leg, pressure, further rubbing, sores and increased swelling made it often difficult to use a prosthetic limb. For Les, the problem was a sinus tract in the flesh at the back of the stump, which became infected and inflamed and required regular drainage until further surgery after two years. Each day, women and men like Bono and Les necessarily address the constraints to, loss of or reduced control over their physical bodies. The dilemma, as they recognized it, is that the physical impairments that compromise bodily integrity challenge their right to recognition, respect and autonomy; their rehabilitative task includes their acceptance and ability to assert their right to social membership.

Most people on whose experiences I draw in this chapter had had amputation. Ian was an exception: his loss of function was due to an aneurysm while he was a graduate student. Ian began his account by describing his loss of full-consciousness, the surrealism of his immobility, the arrival of the ambulance and admission to the hospital, and then the long period of hospitalization and rehabilitation. His memories are vague, and he speaks first of his disengagement from his body in the early days after regaining consciousness in the hospital:

> It seemed like I was looking down a well and through these non-focusing, non-moving eyes, like looking through a lens. But even when

> I talked to myself in hospital in the weeks afterwards, I seemed to be thinking at the back of my mind. I seemed to be talking from a ... maybe I thought the rest of the brain was under siege, entrapped, and this part was the shelter that I'd retreat to or something like that. It seemed to me that I was talking to myself from the back of my mind, from the back of my skull, I don't know why, that's what it seemed to be.

From this memory of dissociation and dislocation, Ian turned to describe his experience of rehabilitation. This is a period he characterized as a one of intense focus and resistance. Ian responded to his doctor's prognosis with a fierce determination to prove him wrong:

> I remember a doctor a few days later came up to me and said, um, told me that I'd never walk again. And I thought "yeah ok." After a couple of days with the right hand side of my body not moving, basically we were going to start all the therapy, I just said "I'm going to do every therapy you want me to." ... I thought, well, I realized, that everything the staff were doing was designed to help me, so I would cooperate to my fullest extent. I was just, you know, "Give me more therapy, I'll just keep going." I didn't despair, I just worked out that, I'd sort of convinced myself that if I worked hard, that I'd get better. Well, even though I knew that I wouldn't be the same person, I only really had a foul day or a black day on a couple of days.... I didn't get depressed. And I just seemed to know that doing therapy would help and in fact I wanted to do more therapy and I got the speech therapist to give me homework and sat in bed trying to do that, I had to learn the alphabet again and then to write the alphabet but I also wanted to do more physiotherapy.

Ian was convinced that the harder he worked, the more likely he would regain function and so the sooner he would leave the hospital. He was initially uncomfortable with using various assistive devices to grip to open doors, pick up items that he could not take up by hand, and so on, but he learned to use them, he explained, because the cost of not using them was far greater:

> In my thoughts over the couple of years since being in hospital and using these devices, I became aware, through not taking them out to dinner and being caught short and then having to get someone else to cut my things, I felt social embarrassment and my independence was threatened. I became aware that all these things really are items of independence and they have a very powerful place in my, like, soul,

in me. So then I met other people who have relationships with their devices, it is just them. When I was growing up, too, a friend of mine had an artificial leg. He'd lost his leg when he was 14 in a motorcycling accident and he had a good sense of humor and like, he'd go camping and he could break firewood over his leg. So I just became adjusted to the fact that these items were essential, and that was so good.

Ian therefore drew on examples of other people who had dealt with bodily change to think about his body as a tool, objectifying and reconfiguring it to incorporate orthotic devices and aids into daily habitus – in his words, his soul. Ian speaks of learning to walk again while a rehabilitation inpatient and in doing so, of becoming far more aware of others' walking: "I became very, very observant of other people's gait. I'll look and see other people that might have a slight limp or they're doing something slightly strangely – and the thing that really surprised me was how many people in the outside world had something wrong with their gait, something out of the ordinary." Because Ian has foot drop, he walks with a cane, and walking involves mindfulness:

> The foot drops and I have to wear [orthotic] shoes. Well, I can walk around the house [without the shoes], but if I walk outside I have to because it [the foot] drags. And so many times, I've actually bent the toes under and really hurt them, and like, while I've lost the first level of sensation, I still have middle pain and highest pain. If I stand on something, like a rock, most people move their feet but I just put more weight onto my feet, and suddenly I get this signal that there is a lot of pain there. I haven't run since [the aneurysm]. I walk very fast but I won't break into a stride or a run because of not knowing exactly where the foot is and I'm not quite sure whether it's going to land on the ground like this or like that. I think mainly it's the pain that's associated with it – I don't run. That's the one thing, because everyone runs in their childhood, but I'm too scared to run. I'm not going to take that risk. Because when I was learning to walk again, this foot, I tripped myself up several times and it [foot] goes in between the legs and so yeah, the pain and the injuries I've done – that's why I don't do it. I was taught by pain.

Ian's hand presented even greater problems: a craftsman, he worked with his hands. Thirteen years on, he still dealt with the difficulties of work by objectification and self-consciousness:

This hand has dropped dead – like, I mean, to open the door, I have to put more clawing into this hand and, I mean, I have to look at my hand so that I can see that physically it closes, and then I have to open it to take the key, and I have to go "there's something in there, there's something in here, there's something in there, don't drop it, don't drop it, don't drop it, don't drop it, don't drop it," and as soon as I start thinking about other things – "bang" – that pisses me off. More than anything it's the hand that pisses me off. Well, it doesn't really piss me off, I accept it, but it annoys me. When I've wanted to do something, it betrays me and drops things. Or sometimes when I might be carrying that [pointing to a book] around and then I start doing something and forget that I'm carrying it. And sometimes it [hand] actually holds things, so I'll be walking like ten minutes and look down and I'm still holding something. And it's like I said, I was wanting to go through the door and I had to hold this book and I was trying to open the door and for a minute I stopped for my hand to hold onto the lock, and it [hand] dropped it [the book] and it's damaged the spine, and I just went *Aaaaaarrrgghh* and I bit my hand: Take that, you mongrel! I'd never done that before – just the FRUSTRATION!

Figure 3.3 Prosthetic arm; 1850–1910. Steel hand and forearm and leather upper arm. Courtesy of Wellcome Library, London.

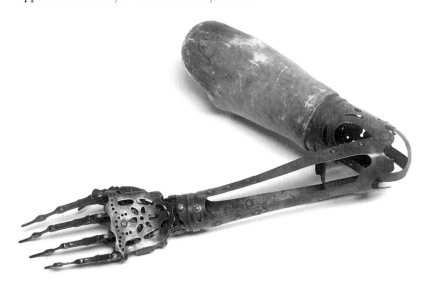

In this extract, Ian graphically illustrates his objectification of the hand affected by his aneurysm. His hand is *it* not *me*, its incapacity to respond according to his intent is imagined as an instance of its willful resistance. The hand pisses Ian off; he bites it to punish it.[1]

Ian also had residual communication, cognitive and interactional difficulties: some aphasia and apraxia, difficulties in being in crowds, using the telephone and understanding numerals (e.g. phone numbers). But he is pragmatic, articulate and insightful about the relationship between the social environment and his communication difficulties: "It's hard to explain to people and the worse problem I have is actually talking to people on the phone. Normally I look at people's faces and their mouth and the context or the situation and if a word is a bit blurred, I can just work it out." He finds it difficult to translate ideas to written text, but he rationalizes this both by drawing an analogy with what is now an 'ordinary' common learning disorder (dyslexia) and by finding precedence in his own life: "I was a terrible writer anyway. I could write, but I didn't like doing it." Multiple other negative effects have been set in place, too: Ian's reading habits have changed but as he tells it, for the better; he enjoys music less, but regards this as a minor change of habit. His craftwork has changed from small-scale constructed pieces to working with different media in large form, and to teaching. This is re-evaluated in terms of artistic maturity rather than as an outcome of a physical constraint. Ian sees his new work as more 'polished,' and he finds support for his shifts in style, material and composition by reflecting on his prior experiences and interests:

> I am more staid in my work now; I used to be freer, more spontaneous. Now maybe because things take a lot longer to get them to fruition, then my style is very structured, not overworked, but very polished, I suppose, very exact. Like I said, beforehand I used to do a lot more spontaneous work, now I don't. The thing that worried me was losing my hands, me not having two hands, and I hadn't worked out what I was to do. It was only when I'd been in hospital for about three months that they introduced me to the one handed clamp. I started using it; they had a little workshop there and I was allowed in there, under supervision, and once I had the one-handed clamp everything became ... ah, I can actually hold things. Ah, there's an option. And I've always liked power tools. I must admit when I left school I worked for three years in a joinery, a factory, I was actually employed in the office but anytime that they needed extra help on the factory floor, I'd

race down and help them for the rest of the day and I actually loved it and so I already knew a lot about industrial woodwork and machines and power tools. The body is a tool. With my body, I have the good side and the bad side.

Body Memories

The body remembers. A photograph evokes images not captured on celluloid, but recalled with other sensory memories: of temperature, sound, smell, taste and emotion. Each new sense opens a shoebox of other indelible memories, not only of people, places and times, but also of perceptions and feelings – fear, sadness and ecstasy that were evoked as part of or by particular experiences. This appears to be particularly so with pain. In their work on trauma, Jenkins and Valiente (1994) reflect on the ways in which bodily memory evokes affect, what Casey (1987) refers to as habitual body memory. For people who experience phantom pain, the body remembers not the affect or emotions associated with the physical loss, although emotion may also be evoked; rather, the brain replicates particular subcutaneous and neural sensations. The phantom life of a limb – the continued kinesthetic experience of the missing body part – is therefore not entirely surprising. Sustained somatosensory and motor maps in the brain allow people to identify the specificity of their anatomy and, as best they can, the valence and quality of the pain.

Around 70 to 80 percent of people who have amputations experience phantom pain to some degree, including episodic pins-and-needles sensations and 'nerve storms' (Hill 1999; Gallagher, Allen, MacLachlan 2001; Flor 2002).[2] Some experience intermittent stump pain or hypersensitivity, and they travel constantly between states with and without pain. At times absorption in another activity can override pain sensation; conversely, pain can flood other states of being, or pain can be the medium through which all other states are experienced (Jackson 1994). The phantom consequently maintains the perception of the integrity of the body long after it has ceased to be so constituted. The neural and somatosensory mechanisms of phantom experience, like other proprioceptive and sensorimotor disorders, such as lack of awareness of deficit (anosognosia) and unilateral spatial and visual neglect, are an expanding field of research for psychoneurology and neurophysiology. Phantom pain and related conditions, including dissociation from the body among individuals with severe

deficits such as hemiplegia or hemianesthesia, as described autobiographically by Oliver Sacks (1984), are relatively well documented. Yet the
manner in which the central nervous system constructs and updates pre-
existing body schema after injury is incompletely understood. Phantom
pain, and the general sense of the presence of a limb that no longer exists,
occurs with amputation when the mental reconstitution of the body is
delayed; the body schema in the central nervous system resists the empirical fact of loss. For people with phantom and stump pain, hypersensitivity
or phantom awareness, the condition is destabilizing and disturbing. Rod,
who lost his right arm and most of his shoulder to cancer, describes the
ever-presence of his amputated right arm as follows:

> I have this phantom arm and it's sitting there. It's sitting across my
> stomach and my mental thought of myself is that I am sitting here
> with you with my right arm across my stomach. It is, well it's not hurt-
> ing or anything, just pins and needles over most of the arm. While the
> phantom arm is sitting there, as far as my nerves, as far as my men-
> tal image is concerned, the arm is there. It's tingling. I'm moving, I'm
> always gesticulating with my hands as I talk, and I'm using my left arm
> to talk to you. And that is my mental image of me.

Rod's missing right arm is actively present because of the sensations of paresthesia. And yet, in terms of everyday embodiment, Rod has
accommodated its absence; he has revised a schema of his body to avoid
automatic uses and prior habitus:

> The worst thing is that if you start to fall, you'll automatically try and
> put out your hand. I don't think I've had that. For me, there's never
> been a frustration because I've tried to put my right arm out to try
> and stop myself and it hasn't been there. I think I've got over that part
> extremely well, almost right from gaining consciousness … it has just
> been automatic. I use my left arm.

Rod speculates that his adjustment derives not as a result of and following the amputation, however, but from a period of immobility prior to
surgery when acute pain prohibited him from using his right arm. And so
he rehearsed its absence. In recalling this, Rod reflects on the difference
between his own experience and that of a person who, following trauma,
awakes without a limb: "The mere fact of having the arm and shoulder off
was no different to the two months beforehand. OK, my body image is
different, but I still can't use my right arm. I've got to do stuff with my left
arm. I had a couple of months, I suppose, to get used to it."

The pain experienced in a limb that no longer exists is confusing for both the person experiencing pain and for others. As Elaine Scarry (1985) highlights, physical pain is phenomenologically complex with respect to its aversiveness, its incomprehensibility, its indescribability and the impossibility for people to empathize precisely with others' pain. Pain is uniquely a feeling without object, preventing people from accessing "an external, sharable world" (5); it has no referential content. It is not *of* or *for* anything, and consequently resists objectification in language. Alfonso Lingis writes of the engulfing and distorting experience of pain, overriding other embodied awareness and mindfulness: "In pain the other sinks back into his or her body.... The flesh in pain is anything but an object; sensibility, subjectivity fill it, with a terrible evidence" (1994:235–236). Ryan explained:

> It's just like pins and needles in your feet really. Most of the time it's just like a phantom sensation. At the moment I can feel the bottom of my foot and my toes are tingling, very slightly. But there's nothing there; it's all in the head. The pain itself is fairly sharp, it's a sharp pain. I can't characterize it. It's like a knife being stabbed into your leg. It's an unnatural pain; it's different. It's memory-driven as opposed to reality. It's a phantom; it's different. Normally they come in the night, when I'm lying in bed, winding down, going over different thoughts, reflecting, doing an appraisal on what you've done in the day and that sort of thing. Your mind goes into a relaxed state and then the phantom pains start coming then. They are only brief, very brief.

The anticipation of pain shapes bodily deportment. Ian, introduced above, spoke of "learning through pain" to use his body mindfully to avoid pain. Phantom pain, however, cannot be anticipated and so avoided. While it is not, usually, experienced in ways that overwhelm and distort consciousness, in other ways, it is frustrating and disorienting for the individual and others in her or his world: indefinable pain in an absent body part. Those who experienced paresthesia regularly found the experience 'annoying' and distressing, as Rod describes:

> From about there through to about there [pointing to the invisible anatomy] it's pins and needles and I'd love to be able to rub it. The other thing that I hate is a really strong gripping pain in the hand – like if I came up to you and suddenly squeezed your hand very, very hard, or grabbed a couple of fingers and really squeezed them hard – I would love to get rid of that. I really would.

Those with phantom pain, and with nerve storms in the residual limb or stump, must learn to live with this nearly incomprehensible experience. Allan recalls:

> Oh pain, now, that was the worst pain that I ever experienced, the nerves coming back in my fingers the following day. That was murder. In general, I judge pain by what I had experienced after the accident and quite a lot of the time if I cut myself or hurt myself I don't even know I've done it because the mind, or subconscious, is judging it on the initial one. But it was terrible and any amputee will tell you how bad that pain is, with the nerves coming back.

Les, in contrast, accepted his surgeon's rather Cartesian view that such pain was 'mind over matter' and he drew on the visual presence of the stump to manage the sensations of the absent limb:

> Even before my leg was amputated, I had spoken to different people and wanted to know what it was like to be an amputee and they said phantom pain, etc., etc. I did mention it to the surgeon who removed my leg and he said to me before my leg was even amputated, the majority of it is mind over matter, and I took that (view) with me away from his office. In the beginning, I guess I did have a bit of phantom pain but I told myself over and over again, I said, don't be stupid, you cannot be having pain in your foot, you don't have a foot, and I just kept telling myself that to the point where it went away.

But later Les returned to reflect on the intensity of nerve pain. Despite his characteristic stoical and dismissive statements, he clearly still experienced extreme discomfort at times, particularly residual limb pain and nerve storms:

> [The pain is] right on the end of the stump, and it can be horrendous sometimes. But I've spoken to my GP about it and he said it's the nervous system and it's very complex and in actual fact, when you do have a part of your body amputated, the nerves are reaching out trying to find their electrical impulse on the other side and when they can't find it, the nerves tie themselves in knots so they can find their … . That's the way he explained it to me, and he explained that when I do get severe nerve pain, that it's probably some of those nerves touching on one another, and he said apart from exploratory surgery to remove that, which I don't want, all you can do is take painkillers when that happens. But as I said, it can be quite severe sometimes. Sometimes it

feels like somebody is actually driving a nail up the end of your bone – that's how severe it can be. But it's very rare. It would happen maybe once every twelve months or so. And once again, I try to put mind over matter and just try to block it out, but it's not always possible when that particular pain is a little too severe for that. But it doesn't affect me emotionally, I guess you'd say, it's just accepting that it's part of being an amputee – all part and parcel.

In contrast, Ryan considered that he had relatively little pain, due to differences in surgery, including the site of the amputation and the degree to which the nerve ends of the stump were protected or exposed. But he also described using a TENS (transcutaneous electrical nerve stimulator) machine to 'soften' the pain. Variously, pharmacology, surgery, electroconvulsive therapy (ECT), electrical stimulation, thermal biofeedback and hypnotherapy were used by participants to reduce pain and related unpleasant sensations. Rod was considering acupuncture, too, in an effort to change his body's schema and so his experience of pain:

> I want to lose the phantom arm because of the problems it's causing – like my doctor does acupuncture and I'm going to see him to see whether acupuncture can be done on me. If it's just on part of a limb that's fine, but with a thing [amputation] so radical, maybe it can't work. But if it can work, and if that phantom arm can be eliminated, I think then my mental image of myself might start to change.

The psychological suffering that accompanies phantom pain can be considerable, and for a number of people, the fear of phantom pain surpassed that of the amputation itself. Lena's ambivalence about whether or not to have part of her foot removed was partly because of her fear of phantom pain: "Oh yes, I could walk a lot further without crutches. But I may gain more pain. Phantom pain's a big issue for amputees. It's variable. I mean, I'd die if I had a phantom pain, if there was a problem like that."

Doing Masculinity

Averted and silenced, the disabled body presents a threat to the very idea of the body, the body in its pure, empty form. It is this idea that informs the prevailing normativities of the body. (Porter 1997:xiii)

The surgically changed, unpredictable or out-of-control body is often assumed by others to be only part of a more extensive disablement, incorporating both mind and body; this in turn threatens the social body. In any cultural setting, people with visible or disclosed communicable diseases threaten the body politic, the social structure and economic footings of society, leading to stigma and exclusion. The breaks of social inclusion and exclusion, stigma and acceptance, are culturally variable, but the perceived threat of social disruption, and consequent stigma, extend to cancer, non-communicable diseases, and other bodily states of being, bodily practice and social identity, including gender identity, sexuality, ethnicity and class. Further, while a person is disabled because he or she may be seen to threaten social order, the processes of stigmatization, in turn, have much to do with the constitution of the disabled body as a generalized threat. As illustrated decades ago, the ill and malodorous, dirty and diseased, odd and ugly are routinely rejected (Goffman 1963; Douglas 1978 [1966]). Leprosy, HIV/AIDS and psychoses provoke rejection because the conditions destabilize at both individual and societal levels, but so, too, do amputation and other physical changes to the body from extreme burns, poliomyletis or kyphosis, for example. Drawing on the experiences of Cambodians who had lost limbs, Lindsay French has argued that others' responses to amputees are visceral, because another's amputation "challenges our own sense of bodily integrity, and conjures up nightmares of our own dismemberment" (French 1994:72). Given the specific context of Cambodia under Pol Pot, French's example demonstrates how terror is imprinted visibly and violently on bodies to control the population. Similarly, acid attacks and burn marks on the bodies of women in South Asia are a shocking reminder of women's subjectivity to men, and control all women's behavior; and few women so assaulted have access to reconstructive surgery to minimize the stigmata of their unruliness or inadequacy (Bandyopadhyay and Khan 2003). Within communities of suffering, the desecration of individual bodies keeps others under subjugation. Far less stigma adheres when bodily flaws do not threaten others, symbolically or literally, and people who have lost limbs conventionally minimize visceral reactions by wearing clothing to cover the stump or prosthesis and harness. At the same time, intermittent media attention to people with disabilities, almost always amputees or people in wheelchairs, both educate and desensitize the public; as I illustrate below, sports successes (through Paralympics and Abilympics, for instance) further reduce negative reactions to certain embodied changes.

The mass media is particularly powerful in setting out common dilemmas and offering viewers (or readers) multiple scripts for social life. For people with impairments, and their families, contemporary films can be read as templates for normalization and reintegration. A number of films use injury and amputation as a central device to explore the existential and relational crises provoked by trauma, as well as using individualized bodily loss as a metaphor for the effects on the national body. Films such as *Coming Home* (Ashby 1978), *The Deer Hunter* (Cimino 1978) and *Born on the Fourth of July* (Stone 1989) build their stories around a central character with paraplegia or amputation, often a war veteran who must now come to terms with loss of conventional masculinity and impotence while dealing with associated and much older psychological scars. *Born on the Fourth of July,* for example, is based on the autobiography of Ron Kovic who, with paraplegia and one leg, returns to the United States from Vietnam to face anti-war demonstrations and his own demons. The dependency is represented stereotypically in these films. Men have lost their autonomy and with this, autonomous sexuality: their sex lives are now characterized as passive and dependent, symbolic, Murphy argues, "of a more general passivity and dependency that touches every aspect of their existence and is the antithesis of the male value of direction, activity, initiative and control" (1987:83). Significantly, in film, the person with the amputation is male, and the amputations are almost always an artifact of war, not from a road traffic accident, misadventure, vascular disease or congenital absence. The loss is heroic and patriotic, and since it is for the nation, it is productive. In consequence the masculinity of the central character is challenged but not fundamentally in question.

Men respond to perceived challenges to their own masculinity by illustrating their determination to normalize their status through conformity, as illustrated in films such as *Murderball* (Rubin and Shapiro 2005). The men who participated in this study were self-conscious of the contradiction of being disabled and male, in terms of the construction of masculinity through social roles and relations, and literally, through the body. They emphasized their role as actors; their priority was to maintain power and control in everyday life. John recalled his early lack of confidence and his continuing frustration with his physical ineptitude in tasks that were (and are) stereotypically men's:

> I did feel that I was going to be rejected by males and females because of my disabilities in the very early days.... In the early days I felt it hard to go and ask the bloke next door to do something for me, change a tap, change a washer, do things I should be able to do. I used to feel very diffident about going and asking someone to come and help me.

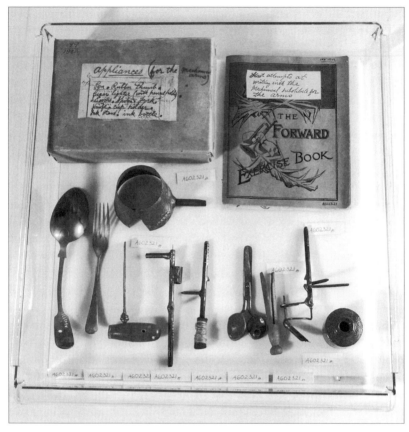

Figure 3.4 Appliances for a WWI "Mechanical Substitute for the Arm."
Courtesy of Wellcome Library, London.

By re-engaging in everyday, masculine-associated pursuits, many men found ways to (re)establish their identity. One man who had lost a leg and an arm, and a number of fingers on his other hand, dressed each day in a shirt and tie as if going to work, even though on a disability pension, to maintain the illusion of being 'useful' if not able-bodied; he drove his children to sporting and other social events to demonstrate his ability to do 'normal fatherly things.' Other men refused to adapt their work routines and practices following surgery, despite family pressure to do so, because this would be 'giving in' to the disease: "I've got to go the extra step in most things," one man explained, "I got to a point where I had to get back to work to get my normality back."

Normality is re-established by returning, as much as possible, to pre-amputation routines, as mapped out for them by rehabilitation goals and practices. Ian's rehabilitation and sense of embodied self arguably were supported by changes in his creative practices, and in the process, by the very masculinity of his new media: "industrial woodwork and machines and power-tools." Other men undertook a range of tasks intended to demonstrate that they were "*doing* as much as the others, *doing* more than my share," and to resist ideas of inequality and dependency. John, again, rejected the idea of being powerless when he needed assistance: "If anything, I feel my disability's given me a degree of power in the way that you can manipulate the situation to your advantage – you can get the benefit. You know they're going to give you the benefit because you're disabled, so that to me was a bit of power." Hence, men often used their prostheses in social contexts to establish their own normality: taking off an artificial leg in a bar or at work to display the device; letting their children take it to school for show-and-tell. John used to be "a bit of a show-off with the hook, do party tricks and things, but that was always good, little fun things like that"; it re-established his position, in Australian idiom, as a "good bloke who could joke with his mates." Les belonged to Sporting Wheelies and participated in competitive weight lifting, and he was also flamboyant, taking off his leg and resting the stump on another chair at work and choosing not to use it on other occasions: "Why should I have to get dressed up to enjoy a barbeque in the backyard or sit down like this? At least I'm comfortable."

Gender and sexuality are unsettled with amputation, and people need to re-establish their adult status. As in filmic representations of amputation, so in the perceptions of the men I interviewed – masculinity, sexuality, sexual attractiveness and performance were complexly and completely entwined. Men spoke explicitly about being sexually active and being able to give and receive pleasure. Amputation is rarely a choice, and the extent to which limb loss might impact on their social and sexual relationships was typically an afterthought and a question that emerged during rehabilitation or subsequently. A few men did have the time to reflect on the possible implications of surgery, however, and they spoke of their concerns about sexual attractiveness when deciding whether or not to have surgery:

> My idea was sort of, "I have to be strong." I am still around a bit longer. I can maybe be around a bit longer. When I actually did lose my leg, I had a girlfriend and she eventually went off to university. At that time,

I had to find myself again and I became more involved with my mates and we went out to parties and things. And I thought, I need to go out and prove that I can get out and meet other women and so forth, as someone without a leg, to find out if women still find me attractive. That is something that I felt I had to get out and do. (Terry)

Other men were concerned especially about sexual function. Allan lost both legs in an automobile accident. His nervousness about re-establishing a sexual relationship with his wife was not because he feared that she would reject him, but because he feared that he would not be able to gain or sustain an erection. And Rod reflected:

It is frustrating to me to be able to use only one hand to touch. I'm a very tactile person. To be able to touch with only one hand, yes, it is a problem – you need two hands to be able to support yourself – so that eliminates a number of sexual positions. Yes, there have been a lot of problems. The problem as far as the arm is concerned I would class as being minor, the erectile problems caused most of the problem. I didn't fear rejection (from his partner) – *that never entered my head* – but I guess I knew I was going to have extreme difficulty in being able to perform the sex act myself.

Conventionally, masculine sexuality and masculinity are defined phallocentrically. Some of the men had erectile dysfunction as well as other functional loss or amputation; for those with vascular disease, this tended to precede their amputation surgery. But asked about sex, men talked of their ability "to give women satisfaction" or, in one case, to "help a woman out," and of being able to pick up women; they saw their amputation as a means to gain attention and sympathy, and they presented themselves as skilled sexual technicians. Les was unmarried when he lost a leg from sarcoma, and he has remained unmarried. He insisted that he was never concerned about his ability to attract women, but he felt that becoming an athlete after the amputation helped him "make it with the ladies." Like other men, he admitted only to some temporary self-consciousness about the stump, "not a fear," he emphasized, "no, but certainly it is there":

It's in your mind. But it's not a fear if you know what I mean. It's not a fear but certainly, I would say something [to a woman], because you don't want to be shocking anybody in that respect, if you know what I mean. But no, I don't think it's made me fearful or anything like that. I'm of the opinion that this is me. If people don't want to … that's their own business, but I don't believe it has affected my approach to anybody or anything that I do. If I approach somebody or I talk to them or whatever and they're not interested [in sex], then so be it. It might be because they don't like the look of me rather than my leg, if you know what I mean.

Les conceded that he went out less often than he might have previously, but he related this to the fact that he had stopped drinking, worked hard full-time, and spent a lot of his leisure time working out at the gym and participating in sporting competitions. Since his involvement in competitive sport followed the amputation, he reasoned that "it's not really to do directly with the fact that I'm an amputee that my social life's been cut in half. It is in the respect that if I were not an amputee, I wouldn't be at the level I am in the sport that I'm in, if you know what I mean." Sexuality, therefore, was only one way through which men saw themselves to be masculine and 'did' masculinity.

Men reconstructed masculinity for personal restitutional purposes through a discourse of normal masculinity, including through rehabilitation programs (Manderson and Peake 2005). Rehabilitation is not revolutionary; as noted earlier, the goal is to enable a person to return to his or her social environment, to maximize function and independence, and to exercise agency and reassert control over the environment. During inpatient rehabilitation and subsequently, individual men sought to re-establish what they understood to be their former relationships with their body, but often they sought to exceed this and to pursue an ideal of hypermasculinity that distinguishes their bodies from those that are feminine, weak and/or sick. The physicality of rehabilitation programs fits with a broader construction of masculinity. Rehabilitation programs for people with paraplegia, Seymour (1998) noted, have successfully drawn on this model to encourage physical activity in exercise regimes, enabling people to lift weights and strengthen their arms to be able to lift their own bodies so as to minimize reliance on others. This has a particular appeal and point of familiarity for men, less so for women, and the men I interviewed were adamant about the importance of physical rehabilitation to ensure that they regained mobility, bodily familiarity and control, and a sense of physical prowess. One man, Simon, reflected on the simplicity of this strategy in enabling him "to get out. I'd gone from pajamas to ordinary clothes and had these crutches":

> It was very important, going through rehabilitation and regaining that feeling of walking again. Taking the first steps. That was sort of a very

unique experience in itself. I had lost my leg. Putting on this artificial leg, walking again, it was such a sense of achievement, to be out there walking again. Standing up, not just sitting down in a wheelchair or standing on crutches. It really was a real sense of achievement. Sort of, you could say, it made me feel one again. You have to adjust and then move on with your life. That acceptance is one step then it goes into adaptation to a lifestyle. You see, you have to adapt to a new lifestyle.

In rehabilitation, men gained an understanding of their present bodily limitations and potential capacity, and of ways to establish a sense of masculine identity concordant with disability. This derived partly from their familiarity with emphasis on physical exercise, as already noted. Many had been involved in sport prior to accident or illness, but even those who were not active had an established interest in sport, a key marker of masculinity within the cultural environment of Australia. In contrast this had little resonance for women, who typically had been much less physically active. Men and women with amputations or functional loss were well aware of the anomalies of gender, and Ryan reflects on this in relation to his own physical practice:

> A lot of masculine things are about power, physical strength, leadership, athletics and the feminine ones would be more along the lines of nurturance and all. [I gained] by getting back into things like sports, leadership positions, and activities that make you feel strong, those things associated with masculinity. Not to say that you forgot you were a man, but to be doing the things that bring a level of comfort, yes, these are the feelings that I like and I want to feel like this. Getting into Sporting Wheelies helped me feel like this. I knew physical fitness was going to be an issue for me. You know, I was just a big bloke naturally anyway. I knew I had to make the extra effort now to maintain reasonable fitness, and the only option I had was to go and work out in the gym. It was important to me to be the muscliest bloke in the gym. I felt that I always wanted to look like the perfect bloke: huge biceps and chiseled chest. I mean that was what was cool. And I had to work on that and I did. I had to see that I maintained my weight and when I got in the gym, I discovered that I could really make it bigger and better than it was. I mean, I worked out in the gym for two years straight, five days a week. Pumping iron. I got pretty solid and pumped out. I would go out and the chicks were like, you know, magnets.

The success that men enjoy within disability sports is not transferable, however, and lacks the power to transform men's primary status from patient to sporting hero. But the men with whom I spoke shared a perception of the uniqueness of their achievements and had other ways of taking meaning from it. In particular, men drew on a discourse of normality; they reclaimed their masculinity either by establishing their athletic competence through re-involvement in prior activities such as swimming, or by joining sporting associations and programs designed to address their specific needs and new capabilities (e.g. the Sporting Wheelies Association, Paralympics, etc.). Sport enabled men to experience their bodies as vehicles of agency and control: "It makes you feel whole again, like I am a whole person. You can actually do something. You are not just stuck in the house. You can do something." At the same time, by joining a community group associated with a particular activity, men were able to forge a normal identity within a community of sameness. In Judith Butler's terms (1990), this is doing masculinity; men could perform their identity. But it also enabled them to build social capital (Woolcock and Manderson 2009), as Simon explained, "building on the male bonding process, going out with the fellows, having a few laughs" to "get back into what society deems to be normal," to recover and redefine masculinity:

> Yeah, definitely feelings of hope and being normal, but also feelings of – you don't have to fall into what society deems to be normal. You can go out and do this wheelchair sport which is the closest thing I have found to football – getting you back into your normal sporting and recreational life. Yes, it is really getting that competitiveness back from sport. It [the lived experience of being] really comes back to sport, I find, more than anything. Just getting out there and having a go. It is really good fun. People really love it. Your teammates are there. It is a real bonding, social experience. But, if I look deeper, then yes, it is me getting out – getting into something else and enjoying it, definitely getting out there and pushing yourself to the limit and seeing what your limitations are but then also trying to beat that bloke who has done all these marvelous things. You want to be better than him! That testosterone drive that keeps you wanting to play, wanting to push the boundaries further. It is something like learning to be acclimatized, or rather, to be comfortable with their disability. It is very important with regards to the body image they are presenting.

Simon refers to the social enactment of masculinity, what Connell (1995) refers to as the "pleasure of sociability" through shared activity. Simon also reflects on how everyday interactions among men provide them with ways to gain self-confidence and affirmation, regardless of injuries or disease that set them apart. In the company of other men, men learn, too, to be comfortable with their prosthesis and to joke about bodily limitations; they spoke of affirming moments over a pint of beer, "mucking around with the other blokes."

A Normal Life of Sorts

Physical components of rehabilitation therefore support men's steps to reclaim identity. Men see themselves as actors, and their own rehabilitation projects are ones of action and activity. Men do masculinity. In contrast, women's usual experience of the body is passive. Berger, some decades ago, argued that a woman "is almost always accompanied by her own image of herself," and accordingly "she comes to consider the surveyor and the surveyed within her as the two constituent yet always distinct elements of her identity as a woman" (1972:46–47). Positioned already as object and Other, women must integrate into their images of themselves the changes to the structure and function of their bodies, and match this new image with and against cultural constructions of normative femininity that link self-worth and appearance. As I illustrate in subsequent chapters, this is deeply problematic for women who have had stoma surgery or a mastectomy. It was less obviously the case among women who had amputations, regardless of their age. These women talked to a limited extent only about their bodies in terms of appearance and sexuality. Their accounts of disability were dominated instead by three themes: their reclamation of everyday life and activities, their need to be independent, and the emotional costs of disability, in terms of their frustration with embodied loss, loss of function, and the imperative of coping. Women's concerns, prior to and while in the hospital and during inpatient rehabilitation, centered on their ability to continue to meet domestic responsibilities, on how others including their husband (or boyfriend) and children would adjust, and on how they would manage outside the home without drawing on the time and assistance of others. While men talked about limb loss in relationship to their own bodies, women explained it in relation to others. Helen captures the pragmatic responses of most women to amputation, regardless of cause:

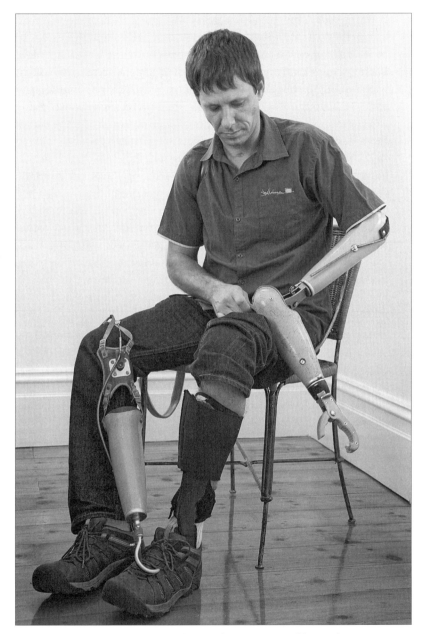

Figure 3.5 Brad Wilkinson, with prosthetic arms and leg orthotic; 2011.
Courtesy of Teresa Gaudio; 2011.

It was a shock, but I knew, nobody was going to chop your leg off unless they've got to do it, you know. I sort of thought, if it's got to be it's got to be, you can't do much about anything like that.... Oh, I think I was worrying about what would happen to me afterwards, what's going to happen to me? You start to think about your leg and about what your life's going to be like and how restricted you're going to be and that, you know. You know, I was determined to be out of there [the hospital] as soon as I could, doing everything they told me to do and trying to do more to help myself. Oh yes, it was like that because I'm not one to sit around and do nothing. I'm on the go all the time, you know, and I was determined to get out of there as fast as I can. [When I came home] I thought I'd be very, very embarrassed by it but it didn't worry me, a look doesn't worry me. All I was worried about was getting around, not what other people were thinking. Well, I feel I'm a lot too old (55) to have to worry about my image, you know, to worry about what I look like or anything. You know, I'm the one who had to walk on it and try and get around on it. It's my body. And if I can handle it, so should everybody be able to.

Other women, although also pragmatic, were more self-conscious of the amputation and limited mobility, and more sensitive to others' attitudes. All women dressed in ways that minimized attention to the prosthetic leg, wherever possible; several talked about conventional feminized acts such as dressing well and having their hair done. Alison, for instance, had lost most of her toes but was reluctant to agree to a full foot amputation, yet also felt stared at and uncomfortable using a walking frame or wheelchair. She began to use an ankle foot orthotic brace to minimize gait problems, and she wore pants to disguise the brace and muscle wastage. Other women initially found it difficult to deal in public settings with curious stares and occasional insensitive comments, and battled with the conflicts that emerged in terms of their physical ability, sense of self, and the attitudes of other people:

> I'm learning to get over it and I'm not taking any notice of it. You feel different and you see people take a side look at you and then look again. And that doesn't bother me because I think they're probably thinking, poor soul, no legs. But you don't want their pity. You want their help. No, I'm not one scrap different to you, only I haven't got your legs. That's the only difference, you know. They don't know how to treat you or what to say. That's the problem for me. I had a feeling

that people think there's something wrong with you when you're disabled or something; you can see the look on their faces, you know.
Mentally you're still the same person. I used to think, oh I won't be
able to do this, but then I thought, no, that's the wrong attitude, I will
do it. I'm still the same person. And it's not what you can't do, it's what
you can do. (Jean)

Jean articulates the nature of impairment and the contradictions that
it produces for individuals, while emphasizing that disability is socially
produced through interactions of the individual and the social environment. Other people, as she makes quite clear, put disability upon her. But
Jean is also mindful of the meanings of the body for the owner of the body
and for others in society. Fisher (1990:18) has reflected that "human identity cannot be separated from its somatic headquarters in the world. How
persons feel about their somatic base takes on mediating significance in
most situations." Cultural esthetics shape perceptions of physical bodies.
The links between physical embodiment and self-perception dominate the
concerns of some people in this study whose bodies fall within the 'normal
range,' as in society more generally. Such values influence people's sensitivity to and ideas about the alignment of physical, cognitive and moral
attributes, and shape interactions with others. Hence Jean's comment that
people extrapolate from physical to mental status, and her insistence, in
response, that "I'm still the same person." But Jean also felt that it was easy
to over-interpret people's awkwardness in social contexts, and she considered that the person with the impairment should take responsibility for
this: "You do feel left out sometimes. But then that's really your own fault.
Because you should join in their conversation and win yourself over and
join in whatever they're doing if you can."

Bono spoke in similar ways as she rationalized other people's attitudes
and her adaptation:

Well, like, one time we were going to go to a party and people said,
oh well, if she feels embarrassed about coming, we'll understand. But
I wasn't embarrassed. You know, other people are embarrassed, not
me. They used to say to me; aren't you worried about the legs? I'd say I
can't worry about the legs; I haven't got them anymore. I'm not going
to spend my whole life worrying what happened to my legs just
because I haven't got them. I can't put them back. I can't do anything
else about it; if they're gone they're gone, that's it. I've got to get up and
get on with my life. I can't just sit by.

Several women observed that others see people with disabilities differently, and they commented on the importance that they distance themselves from attitudes of pity, curiosity, and occasionally hostility. Even so, women almost uniformly drew on common cultural constructions of normalcy to situate their loss of mobility, in order to 'lead their own lives.' While Lena spoke of detaching herself from the fact that she had had a foot amputated, she did so to avoid feeling overwhelmed by it, "Some days I pretend I'm perfectly normal." Other women did not *pretend* they were normal; they *were* "just normal women with one leg." Women viewed their problematic body and its appurtenances – the stump, the prosthesis, orthotic brace, wheelchair, crutches or walking stick – as contradictory or irrelevant to their state of being normal. They were irritated when people treated them as disabled. In this insistence, women sought to separate corporeality and self, to break an assumed interdependence of the body and the self. In women's own words, they were each "just the same person ... wanting to just do normal things." Such normal things were mundane, everyday activities, aspects of their ordinary life pre-surgery that contributed to their social identity:

> I want to do just normal everyday things like go to the toilet myself, do a bit of cooking, washing up, things like that, for myself. I don't want to sit in a wheelchair the rest of my life. And like your bodily functions don't work as well, or anything. At least if you can move around a little bit. That's why I thought I might be able to keep my leg, the second leg. (Julie)

> At first, I felt useless. Then as time went past and I learned to do things, I thought, well, I'm not so useless. You feel that you're not the same person, but you are the same person – it's only the fact that you haven't got that leg or legs, whatever it might be. You've just got to get yourself into normal habits with what you've got left and that's all there is to it. And not say, poor me, I haven't got legs. (Jean)

Women were frustrated at times by the contradictions between their own goals and interests and their inability to do all they wanted, and frequently reflected on their loss of control over how they used their bodies, of the implications of this in terms of choice, freedom and autonomy, and their dependency on others. Women who rated freedom highly were suddenly faced with the implications of their loss of mobility: "Apart from the inconvenience and the limitations on my lifestyle, I can survive and I can cope quite well. But it's limiting. It limits my job and my mobility is too limited to do a lot of different things. I have to be committed to this job because there aren't too many options" (Lena).

Women who prized their autonomy felt that their lives had been 'completely turned around' or that they had been 'stopped in their tracks,' and they were restricted in the number of things they could now do. Women who had a strong sense of competence felt undermined; those who saw themselves as independent had to adjust to their activities, expectations and their relations with others, at times choosing not to undertake a particular activity to avoid creating further dependency. Bono was particularly articulate here:

> I get frustrated because I can't do what I want to do. I look at things and I think that should be done, you know, because I'm so used to always doing it, you know, pre losing my leg. And like the frustration gets bad because you just, if you have been a very active person it's *like cutting your legs off*, and you just can't go anywhere. I feel a lot better when I'm able to walk around and move around a bit. There are times when you want to do things. That's normal in everyday life, you know. Normal people do that. But you cope, and that's the main thing I suppose – just cope with these things, be able to go from day to day, I just live from day to day now. If I get through one day, good – carry on. I think mentally I'm strong in that department. I do get a bit upset as I say, but most of the time I'm very positive about things.

This says nothing of how others relate to those whose bodies are injured or malfunctioning. Fear of rejection lay at the heart of the insecurities of many people who had undergone major surgery or sustained permanent injury. However, while women were articulate about their everyday lives, their need to re-establish order, and the frustrations, in contrast to men, they were relatively reticent about intimacy and sexuality, bodily change, sexual confidence and lovemaking. Their sexual and personal relationship status varied. Some women were no longer sexually active. Others resumed their sexual lives and saw accommodation as technical rather than emotional or esthetic, adopting a different position in sexual intercourse, for instance, to reduce discomfort. Jean tended to see sex post-surgery as a matter resolved through communication, and reflecting dominant views of gender relations and behavior, blamed other individual women for specific difficulties: "You learn to get over these things. You've got to learn to do these things. I can see that it could make a big difference in a marriage if you withdrew. But it's not the amputation, it's the woman turned away, feeling sorry for herself and wanting to be pitied." Other women, however, worried that the amputation and limited mobility, and the need for greater care, would impact on sexual and other dimensions of their relationship with their partner. Kay put it this way:

> Well, I think it's all in the mind. I've had some very, very bad days. When I first came home, I would cry at the drop of a hat. But that is part of healing. This is the loss of a part of your body. When I was thinking about having my leg amputated, I was worrying, what's it going to do to our marriage? I never thought I'd have to have my husband to shower me or do those sorts of things. That's what really worried me. It takes your dignity and everything away. I know you lose dignity when you have children, but when your husband's got to do your toileting.... But I'm still a whole person as far as I'm concerned. My husband thinks I'm a whole person, so that is the main thing. He didn't turn away. And it's not like having a breast off; I can't imagine having a breast off. The only thing that's gone is my leg. The mind hasn't gone.

Younger women without partners were particularly cautious of sexual involvement. Alison was seeing someone when she was participating in the study, but had not yet established physical intimacy: "I have my moments, but on the whole, feeling secure in the friendship is really important and just knowing who I am, just being secure within myself, is most important now." Lena recounted how she withdrew from her previously regular social activities following her amputation, and had to make an effort to "go out and socialize." She found it difficult to engage intimately in any way post-surgery, and was very anxious about establishing a sexual relationship:

> Even though it had never, never happened before, I shut out even the possibility of ever picking a guy up and bringing him home for the night – not that I ever would have done it before, but I thought it would be really difficult now to explain to someone that I didn't know ... that I didn't have [a foot].

She finally became involved with someone after a year, with a man who was "very gentle...very tender about it and a very liberal sort, and it didn't worry him at all and so I had a very fulfilling sort of physical relationship with him."

Losses of Function

Differences in mobility and independence among participants were substantial, affecting their employment, personal relationships and social engagement. In this section, I explore the experiences of those who had extensive loss of function without amputation, as may occur with severe stroke or spinal cord injury. These men and women faced a complex task of negotiating bodily loss and change, and their accounts of disability, rehabilitation and adaptation provide further insight into the multiple ways in which, through narrative, people interpret their experiences to re-assert control over their own lives. Robyn, for example, was a young woman who had broken her back in a fall from a horse. In four months of inpatient rehabilitation, her tasks focused on using a wheelchair and learning alternatives to taken-for-granted bodily skills that date from early childhood: learning to dress herself, for instance, "to move around and transfer from a bed onto a chair and a bath seat onto a chair and all that kind of stuff." But this was the starting point only, one that Robyn shared with any person who loses mobility or function:

> I learned things a lot better when I got home, how to do things, and you know, there'd be things you come up against at first and you think, "Oh, my God, how am I going to do this?" and then you find a way to do it. So, you know, it's a good feeling because you've found your own way to do that, and I still work out how to do things now. You're coping with things like the fact that your bowels and bladder aren't working properly any more, and they train you to deal with that. But you have to deal with the fact that during time in hospital your bowels are out of control. You have to learn how to deal with it. A lot of people wear catheters, they wear tubes with a bag for their urine for their bladder, you know, for the rest of their life, or they have some other kind of catheter arrangement. I didn't have to. I found if I compressed my abdominal muscles I could empty my bladder, so I can do that. Catheters – if I ever have a catheter, I get a urinary tract infection. To move your bowels, you have to learn how to deal with that, too – people have different patterns of bowel motions and every morning, every second morning, so you can't have an accident.

Post-surgery, Robyn, like others with continence problems, has had to map her physical environment and shape her activities around personal bodily contingencies:

It's organization, you know. When you've got a disability, especially in places that don't cater very well, you have to organize in advance a lot. You have to think, "If I go to that shopping center, I can't go to the toilet, but if I go to that one I can go to the toilet, so I'll go to that one after that one, but I can't go to the post office at that one so I'll have to go to this one."

In recounting her adjustment, Robyn repeatedly turned to the assumptions that other people tended to make about her ability and interests, to do things for her without consulting, anticipating her needs. Robyn interpreted such actions as a presumption by others that they knew what was best for her, and she reflected that such attitudes stripped her of a sense of competence: "I'm actually very independent and I hate people doing things for me and people do try and do things for you more than is actually necessary because they think ... everyone with a disability is so different, everyone has a different degree of disability." Robyn also reflected on the need to distance herself from overprotective or invasive behavior:

If you worried about it all the time, you'd go mad, you know, sometimes you can't help it because people do tend to stare at you a bit. Yeah, yeah, you feel you don't want people to stare back. It was hard because I hadn't had these experiences all my life. I mean, of course, I worried about it, and I felt fat and all that kind of thing. But people's emotions get thrown at you when you've got a disability, you know, you get "Oh, you poor thing," and the staring and so on, and you just have to cut off after a while because you'd go mad if you noticed it all. You just have to cut off and lead your own life.

Dominant community attitudes about the homogeneity of experience of disability and the common limits to function and mobility informed other kinds of social interactions, including presumptions about the desirability of particular kinds of social interaction: "People have a strange idea that because you've got a disability you hang around with other people with disabilities." Robyn's housemate asked her not to return to their shared apartment when she left the hospital, a few of her friends stepped back, and she required union support to end harassment from a work supervisor unconvinced of her competence. She worked hard to maintain her involvement, informally and formally, in worlds of work and leisure that did not center around, and so center her identity on, her wheelchair: "I guess I don't want to fit into the stereotype of, you know, somehow, you know, just all be in a little group together with other people with disabilities." She also had to deal occasionally with overt discrimination: "If people put me in a bad situation, I don't feel as though I have to accept that, you know, I feel like I can fight back, and – and use whatever rules or whatever (mechanisms) there are to assist me."

Negative social attitudes undermined Robyn's sense of sexual agency in particular. During hospital-based rehabilitation, men were more likely than women to ask questions about the impact of their bodily change on their sexuality and on sexual function, confidence and lovemaking. Robyn related this both to the greater visibility of sexual dysfunction in men, and "the whole thing with men about their virility and their maleness and all that, coming out through the physical self." She suggested that "women are used to being more flexible" and able to adjust to social and embodied changes. But her reflections on her own experience suggested that this was not necessarily the case. As an adolescent, Robyn was self-conscious, partly due to "bad propaganda" from her mother, who told her "that [she] was too tall to ever get a man" (175 cm, or 5'9"). In the hospital after the injury, immobile, Robyn gained weight and felt "fat and ugly." Nurses were evasive when she asked them directly about sex and sexuality, other than in the most general and allusive terms (the possibility of having a baby); this contrasted with how she (and male participants) perceived nurses' willingness to acknowledge and manage men's sexuality during rehabilitation: nurses took men out of the hospital occasionally, and "married them and things like that." Robyn's doctor was "abrupt and tactless."

> I didn't know what would happen; I didn't think I'd be acceptable to anybody. Then this doctor, he said to me one day: "Oh well, do you want the bad news now? Have you got your razor blades ready? Women with disabilities, you know, don't have as good a time as men with disabilities because, you know, men find it harder to deal with disability than women do. Women are nicer, women are more understanding and caring and all that sort of thing."

Robyn did not think that her accident had significantly affected her sexual desire or responsiveness, and she described herself as having a strong libido. Yet she did not become romantically involved with anyone for several years after the accident, and she explained this extended period of celibacy as due to her own lack of confidence. While Robyn was wary of establishing a sexual relationship because of her doctors' comments to her, she reflected on her own perception of men's alleged predatory attitudes towards women with disabilities, as she understood from other people with amputations: "The whole thing with sexuality, the whole thing on the Internet, there's all these people who are actually turned on by people with amputations, and there's all these sites on the Internet, people trying to link up with people who are amputees." These negative social attitudes and practices were recursive. Robyn's first sexual relationship occurred some years after her accident with a man who proved unstable, volatile and abusive; the relationship continued for some time because she felt power-less and dependent. Her current happier relationship is with a man with a mild physical disability, and she was pleasantly surprised when she began the relationship: "I think I'm probably a bit defensive. I'm – I'm – yeah, a bit more cynical. I didn't expect people to find me attractive because of my disability, but he seems to, and I believe him, you know, so yeah, it's just different ways people look at you." Through her lover, she has become involved in disability activism, in the process gaining greater personal resilience, and also, as she reflects, "a realization that all sorts of physi-cal bodies can be attractive to some people.... I mean it's a matter of how you look at people, and people have all got different things that they're attracted to physically as well as in terms of personality, you know. I think the more you like a person the more attractive they look to you anyway; you know, they come to look more attractive to you."

Troubled Terrain: Amputation in Film

We use bodies as vehicles of expression. We enact thoughts, ideas and emotion, and we interpret other bodies in this light. People's claims of being 'normal' derive from their sense of normalness in relation to state of mind rather than body, but this is influenced by how others consider the two to merge. The body may reflect the state of the mind either through simple analogy, or as a causative, corporeal difference diverting the course of the mind. Obvious physical differences bring the relationship of body and mind to the foreground.

The extraordinary Japanese film *The Face of Another* (1966) exposes this tension between surface and self, and the psychopathology of loss. The film begins with an X-ray vision of a man, the facial bones moving as he describes the industrial accident in the plastics factory that led to his disfigurement. Okuyama (Tatsuya Nakadai) is profoundly scarred, his face all but destroyed. He wears bandages over his face and head, with space only for his eyes and lips. He is bitter and vengeful; he ruminates on destroying his wife's face, or gouging out her eyes. "The face is the door to the mind," he explains to her. "Without it, the mind is shut off. There's no communication. The mind's left to corrode, to disintegrate. The mind of a rotten monster." His psychiatrist convinces him to wear a mask rather than impose on himself isolation or death. They choose a face from an unknown man in a coffee shop. The mask is made in the psychiatric clinic, a space that is adorned with prosthetic ears, da Vinci's Vesuvius Man, a wooden drawing manikin, and glass etched with Langer's Lines, ellipsoidal lines that may be mapped onto the skin to correspond to the orientation of collagen fibers (Figure 3.6). With the mask and so a new face, new clothes and a new apartment hidden from his wife, Okuyama begins to live a second life propelled by his desire for revenge. He seduces his wife; he assaults another woman. Released from custody, he stabs his psychiatrist fatally.

Faces are perhaps a special case; limbs can be overlooked, ignored, or worked with. And many people find ways to re-establish their lives and their self-identity by techniques and technologies of resistance. People with wheelchairs have no option other than to work with the technology; the chair precedes them in their interactions with others. Similarly, functional hand prostheses are difficult to disguise, more so than is true for

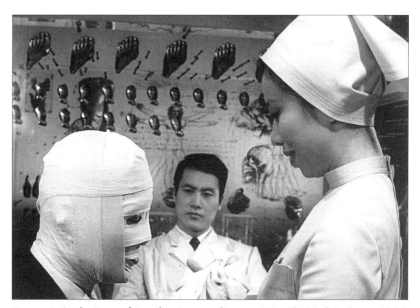

Figure 3.6 *The Face of Another,* Japan, director Hiroshi Teshigahara; 1966. Courtesy of Photofest.

prosthetic legs or feet if hidden by trousers and boots; hands then also prefigure in social interactions. But most limb prostheses, because they are external to the body, are visible, and their use requires considerable intentionality for the wearer, at least at the outset, as he or she adapts his or her body to use the technology, develops muscle strength, shifts position and varies action to enable its integrated habitual use. External, removable prostheses and orthoses become thematically central and integrated into the body through practice.

As described in the previous chapter, not all people who use prostheses do so in ways that ensure that the technology is peripheral, nor are they worn in discrete ways to minimize difference and enable normality in action and interaction. Some people use or refuse to use prostheses and other devices performatively, underscoring bodily change or loss, so finding an alternative way of exercising agency and, therefore, rejecting the social construction of normal. As illustrated by broadcasting journalist Kath Duncan, in her film *My One-Legged Dream Lover* (Duncan 1999), while prosthetics design has advanced to maximize the 'life-like' appeal and appearance, amputees may refuse to wear a cover over the prosthetic spine (an aluminum or carbon fiber tube) or refuse to wear clothes that disguise a prosthesis; they may instead wear shorts or a skirt that exposes it, and/or use a prosthesis that by design advertises the bodily absence. In doing so, people insist on a personhood that is contingent neither on surface nor (apparent) corporeal integrity. Women concurrently challenge the social construction of gender. Further, by making visible the scars of disease or injury, such embodied decisions destabilize social illusions of a healthy society. Pete, who lost a leg from an osteogenic tumor, explained:

> It doesn't bother me, my artificial leg. I don't have a prosthetic cover on it. It is completely metal. People might be looking at me when I walk around or whatever, but hey, this is me, I am walking around here doing my own thing. If they want to have a look, then feel free. I am comfortable with it so. It's a way of putting it out there. I may be more extroverted than introverted wanting to put myself out there – more being a person with a disability rather than just a person. In everyday life, I still see myself as the same person though, perhaps just a bit more extroverted. I have to put myself more out there – any achievements you can get across.

Pete is an exception, however. A key to why men and especially women focused on the normalness of appearance, as well as how they live their lives, lies in the further analysis of resistance.

Some of this resistance takes place in the context of disability activism, some in relation to the selection of prosthetics. The company Otto Bock (Germany), for instance, produces patterned and multi-colored cases for prosthetic limbs, lifelike in proportion (length and width) but without the illusion of fleshiness. Prosthetic technicians, even in small clinics, increasingly make their own cases, personalized for their clients. Sporting prostheses are often flamboyantly unlike fleshly limbs. One might argue also that both amputee 'devotees' (people with acromotophelia) and 'wannabees' (people with apotemnophilia) create resistance to dominant sexual mores, although many people who have congenital limb abnormalities or are amputees from injury or disease are uncomfortable with or disturbed by these two groups of (primarily) men (Duncan and Goggin 2002). Within heterosexual constructions of sexuality (little is written of homosexual desire in this context), the former (devotees) are men attracted to women with amputations – the stump is fetishized. The latter (wannabees) are men and very occasionally women who want to become amputees themselves and may seek surgery to this effect. Disability activist groups make a finer distinction between devotees and fetishists. Devotees are explicit about their sexual attraction to the amputation. They may place themselves in situations, working in sporting events for people with disabilities or in prosthetic or rehabilitation facilities where they can interact with amputees and touch the limbs, but they are constructed as 'safe' because of their openness. Amputee fetishists, on the other hand, are constructed as "extremely dangerous."[3]

This says little about the self-esteem and body image of men and women without limbs, and claims of being 'normal' need some further interrogation. I use as my example the film by Australian radio journalist Kath Duncan, self-described as a 'double congenital amputee' (LBE, RAK – that is, left below elbow, right above knee, defining the terminal points at amputation). In the treatment prepared for the film,[4] however, Duncan represented herself (ironically) as a woman born with Facial Limb Disruptive Spectrum, with one full right arm and one full left leg. The film, *My One-Legged Dream Lover* (Fowler-Smith and Olsen 1999), documents Duncan's visit to the United States from May to July 1998, including her interactions with amputee devotees. When the treatment was written, Duncan had "a very low tech artificial leg which works by vacuum suction" needing to be replaced on a three year basis; the treatment indicated that in the U.S., she would "be shopping around for a new leg and the latest in arm technologies." In the treatment, too, the film was described as "an achingly funny and provocative film about the body, the mind and desire." In effect, it focused particularly on the latter (desire), bringing to the fore "the troubled terrain that divides one body from another, one life from another, a gender, a culture, from others" (Duncan and Goggin 2002:131). Many of the proposed scenes were excluded. The final version of the film offers poignant insight into why people with amputations stress normalcy, and why they use conventional gender roles to illustrate this to the world at large.

My One-Legged Dream Lover begins with underwater footage of Duncan swimming, her fleshy body and irregular limbs exposed; she is playing with the freedom that water offers us all. In the voice-over, she speculates: "If I told you there was a place you could be completely adored, just for who you are, wouldn't you wanna go there? If you had to cross oceans to get there, wouldn't you wanna try? If you could make your most secret fantasies come true, how could you resist?" The following scenes provide context: Duncan speaking by phone to an amputee fetishist, Duncan searching the worldwide web, putting on her leg prosthesis, sitting at her desk and explaining why most of the photographs on the wall are of herself: "I put up photos to remind myself that I still exist and that I'm not that weird." She explains why she is curious to meet amputee devotees and to attend the Fascination meeting: "I don't want to be victimized, but it's power I've never had. I don't mind playing to it."

Her first meeting with devotees is at Venice Beach, California, where she meets with two men with whom she had communicated by email. She is curious about their willingness to share with her their photograph collections, porn videos (*Amputee Holiday, And there were none* ...), comics and ephemera that feed their fetishism: "All of us want 'the real thing' but it's in such short supply." Duncan becomes distraught, not because of their fetishism, but because of the men's comments on other aspects of women's bodies and their bodily shortcomings – women are judged as too fat, too ugly, or too thin. Duncan feels rejected not because of her limbs, but because of her weight: "I'm upset to find that wherever I go, whoever I'm with, I remain unacceptable."[5] In the chronology of the film, she proceeds to Dallas, Texas, and, captured by "the idea of all of my body being really on display," signs on for a photo shoot of amputee women for devotee consumption. Posing as a warrior princess with a Zulu spear, she is encouraged by the photographer: "You're very special. You have two parts [arm and leg] to present." The distance for women between the social conventions of the body beautiful and the bodies of women lacking limbs is emphasized, as one model explains to Duncan: "It boosted my self-esteem. It makes me feel pretty for just a little while. Like a normal model."

Duncan proceeds to Chicago to attend two annual meetings, held concurrently – one of devotees ('Fascination'), the other, the American Coalition of Amputees, including amputees, various interest groups and prosthetists ('friends') – and Duncan and the crew explore the hostilities of the Coalition towards the devotees, seen as predatory fetishists. They explore, too, the motivation of the devotees, men who "have this thing (desire for a stump) in your belly since you were 6 or 7." Again, Duncan is flattered when the reality of this tension exposes her own lived contradictions: she enjoys being with the devotees – "It's a body thing... you can't ignore the body." But she is distressed by the coalition spokesperson questioning her association with a known devotee as "vicarious righteousness," because the censoring community is her own.

Duncan had planned to replace her prosthetic leg and procure a prosthetic arm; in the end she does neither. But those at the meeting insist on the importance of prostheses in enabling inclusion – "a lot of amputees want to be normal." The price of inclusion is to be mute and to conform, in physical appearance, taste and desire; people find a place in mainstream society by appearing as normal as possible. Duncan looks into the eye of the camera: "The devotees have given up being normal. And so have I." Resisting convention in the film, Duncan is intentionally provocative, wearing garments that make no attempt to hide her limbs, but she is hurt in the process, including especially by those most like her. The liberating experience of attending a meeting with dozens of people who lack limbs, as she does, is immediately stripped from her by her sexual and social choices; these are unacceptable to the majority.

My One-Legged Dream Lover was first screened in Australia on SBS (Special Broadcasting Service) over a decade ago, on April 14, 1999, at the Disability Film Festival in London in 2001, and at other film festivals in Australia, the Netherlands, Estonia, and Canada. Duncan and Goggin (2002), commenting on its reception, note the number of viewers who assumed Duncan was sexually inactive prior to the trip, although given her own comments, in voice-over and directly to the camera/viewers, this was odd. Many saw the film as overtly and offensively sexual. Its promotion prior to its premier screening was a portent of reactions to come, and revealed the discomfort that some people felt about amputee bodies and sexual choice. A letter of complaint led to an enquiry into the promotion and the film itself by the Australian Broadcasting Authority (ABA) (1999), to establish whether the film breached relevant codes of practice regarding sex and nudity, including with respect to the program's bona fides, the responsibility with which visuals and subject matter were treated, the degree of explicitness of visuals, and the impact that visuals had in the context of the program as a whole. The ABA established that the documentary contained voluptuous images of amputees swimming and posing in sexy underwear but no nudity and that, in the context of the program's intent, the images were not gratuitous. It also found that verbal sexual references such as "where do you put your stump during sex?" were discreet and infrequent, and therefore conformed to the PG (Parental Guidance) classification. The authority concluded that children with disabilities of this kind, watching this program in the company of an adult, would have been encouraged by the positive, upbeat message conveyed. It also established that references to fetishism were discreet, and that the described fetish was mild and could not be considered abhorrent. However, although the ABA determined that there had been no breach with regard to sex and nudity, it upheld the complaint that the promotional material shown at 6.30 p.m. contained images and verbal references to fetishism which were unsuitable for children to watch. Specifically, it determined that "images of bulging breasts and women posing provocatively in leather fetish gear, which are edited to give maximum impact, and the verbal references to fetishes and sex" were unsuitable to be shown when children might watch television without parental supervision. The decision arguably had little impact, however, and the film enjoyed considerable critical (although certainly not commercial) success.

But the point was made in multiple ways. The amputated limb is excess not lack, its representation is confronting with respect to the nature of disability, the nature of the individual with the disability, and that of others who interact with him or her. The associations of physical disability with intellectual impairment, the hegemonic notion that people with physical disabilities should be sexually inactive, and the extreme disquiet regarding paraphilia, all reinforce the belief that people with amputation or other visible (surface) anomalies, and those with whom they share their lives, must disguise their disability and establish their normalcy, or remain always on the outer.

These values of the body and disability reflect attitudes to all bodies, and to bodies that are diseased or anomalous. The prescriptions that shaped reactions to Duncan's film – and to Kath Duncan herself – apply equally to any person with a visible impairment or with functional loss. But as I explain in the following chapters, they influence also attitudes to people with health conditions that are obscure to ordinary surveillance. The surface tensions they embody are largely in the minds of those directly affected. But this is enough. Bodies that transgress, that are out of order, create ongoing tensions personally, relationally and culturally.

Notes

1. In the same way that Ian speaks of *it* and *the hand*, not *my hand* or *me*, Lesley Stirling and I illustrate the objectification and distantiation in speech acts of women who have had a mastectomy, who struggle to find an appropriate lexicon to talk about the breast-that-was, the absent breast, the site, the chest and the scar (see Manderson and Stirling 2007).

2. The phantom limb has a long history in provoking psychological, philosophical and surgical reflection. Schilder (1950), among others, suggested that phantom experiences were "an expression of nostalgia for the unity and wholeness of the body, its completion," with variations because of individual differences in emotional reactions to different parts of their body (Grosz 1994; Finger and Hustwit 2003).

3. The website cripworld.com (http://www.cripworld.com/amputee/) has consistently maintained a distinction between devotees (or "admirers") and fetishists in terms of "respect and adult/mature interaction with the amputee." Devotees are characterized as interested in the individuals and open about their motivation, in which the stump serves as an "attraction trigger." Fetishists in contrast are described as reducing the person with an amputation to a "stump" and "prey on new amputees and those with low self-esteem and a negative body image" (http://www.cripworld.com/amputee/devos.shtml, accessed April 16, 2007). Advice at this website in 2003 warned that fetishists were "extremely dangerous and suffering from a severe mental illness and are to be avoided at all costs" (accessed April 30, 2003); more recently amputees have simply been advised of the physical attraction of the stump, and "if you're aware of it and ok with it, then go with your instincts" (April 16, 2007).

4. The treatment was posted at the website of DragonWorks Amputee Connection (http://home.t-online.de/home/Amelo-Forum/hintergrund/theorie2/

duncan3.htm) to ensure that people who might wish to meet Duncan were fully informed of her project.

5. Elsewhere, Duncan comments that she found herself examined under the same close scrutiny in the United States as she did in Australia: "Is she a freak I want or not?" (Duncan and Goggin 2002). Duncan did not find other peoples' rapture in her stumps particularly erotic, but she rejected the construction of the fetishist or devotee as abnormal, a paraphiliac with "a preference for a … less threatening, more attainable or more easily attainable 'love object' for whom the therapeutic task is to return them to normalcy as soon as possible."

4

Body Basics: Living with a Stoma

A disabled body seems somehow too much *a body,* too real, *too corporeal: it is a body that, so to speak, stands in its own way. From another angle, which is no less reductive, a disabled body appears to lack something essential, something that would make it identifiable and something to identify with; it seems* too little *a body: a body that is deficiently itself, not quite a body in the full sense of the word, not real enough. (Porter 1997:xiii) (emphasis in original)*

If this is true for any disabling condition, that the body is both too much and too little, it is particularly so for people whose bodies are impossibly out of control as a result of dysfunctions of the bowel and bladder. Body waste seeps out as liquid and solid, smell and sound, infiltrating space in ways that cause embarrassment to the person and anyone in contact with her. Surgery to rectify this is not always successful, and is only a moment in a prolonged medical and surgical history. Even if successful, still the body exudes; the rustles and flapping of bags, gurgles and belches, odor, leaks and floods continue to conspire against the person and undermine his or her sense of well-being, security and control. People who have stomas can never forget their surgery; they live with the consequent stoma and care for it recurrently each day. Others who have not had surgery but have bladder or bowel problems manage as best they can, attempting to hide the unruliness of their bodies.

Over 2 million Australians are estimated to experience incontinence, although many problems affecting the bowel and bladder are regarded as 'minor.' Urinary incontinence is presented as a 'normal' outcome of childbearing for women, spoken of as 'post-micturition dribble' in men as a 'normal' result of aging and prostate enlargement. Even the mildest loss of urine or feces, the most occasional accident, can be profoundly distressing, however. More serious conditions cause enormous distress. Consider Australian novelist Susan Johnson (1999), and her reaction when she realized that her rectal-vaginal fistula would not heal without a temporary colostomy:

> How do I tell you about lying awake alone in the bed the next night, having discovered my flesh coming apart like rotten fruit, and knowing that it meant a colostomy? How do I transmit to you the fear in my cells, the feeling that my own body was splitting like two halves of a peach? This was the night ... I felt panic scrambling the cage of my chest. I feared that the wall between my vagina and my anus was breaking down, and that by morning I would be left with only one passage out of my lower body, my body's waste cradled in the folds of my vagina. (89)

Because of the general discomfort that people have in speaking about urine and feces, and seeking medical advice on matters relating to the bladder and bowel, community prevalence figures of such medical problems are poor, and relatively little public health attention has been given to them. Morbidity and mortality figures of conditions that result in incontinence and stoma give some indication of the community burden, however. Cancer is a major cause. In Australia in 2010, bowel cancer was the third most prevalent cancer for both men and women (after lung and prostate cancer for men; lung and breast cancer for women), affecting especially people 55 years and older, and was among the ten most common causes of death. Bladder cancer is also relatively common in men. In the United States, colorectal cancer is second most common for both men and women, and bladder cancer is prevalent especially among men over 55. Diabetes mellitus type 2 is increasingly prevalent in Australia and globally, and is a significant risk factor for both urinary and fecal incontinence. Inflammatory bowel disease, diverticulitis and intestinal obstruction are significant conditions in populations in industrialized settings that may lead to surgical intervention, and fecal incontinence from all causes is similar in prevalence in men and women, despite the assumption that obstetric trauma contributes to women's incontinence and that irritable bowel syndrome is also more common in women. Based on various community prevalence studies, urinary incontinence in any population is around 50 percent in women and 25 percent in men over the age of 40, with some increase in incidence with age.

The majority do not seek medical advice for these problems; those who do typically present for care with advanced problems. Approximately 36,000 Australians in 2011, in a population of over 22 million, have a stoma. In North America, possibly a million do. In this chapter, I pursue the everyday experiences and challenges to self-identity that stomas present.

Body Acts

The anus, genitals, and the acts and products of elimination provide small children with endless amusement. As any three-year-old knows without the benefit of psychoanalytic theory, the sound, odor, color, and texture of human waste, and the body parts and settings of evacuation, offer endless possibilities to test parental patience. Speaking about waste is perpetually funny. The most interesting place in a new environment, a shopping center or a fast food restaurant, the first point of call for any pre-schooler, is the bathroom.

Dominique Laporte (2000 [1978]), following Lacan, argues that our attitude towards feces as a source of embarrassment, shame, and pollution is a distinguishing characteristic of humans, and that the management of human waste is crucial to our modern identity, the organization of the city, the rise of the nation-state and the development of capitalism. Notwithstanding that everywhere people are concerned about matter and its place (Douglas 1966), embarrassment regarding feces and defecation is arguably both a cultural and historic construct. Accounts of the everyday life of pre-industrial Europe graphically illustrate the environment of filth and the cavalier disposal of feces in both town and countryside, and as various historians suggest (Corbin 1986 [1982]; Cipolla 1992), the structure of contemporary society around urban and industrial centers would not have been possible without developing systems for the safe disposal of waste. From the mid nineteenth century especially, developments in plumbing and changes in city government enabled night soil to be collected and disposed of systematically, cesspits were covered and emptied, and water closets were introduced. This hygiene and sanitation revolution dramatically reduced the incidence of cholera, typhoid and gastrointestinal disease in these early industrializing societies (Szreter 1988; Gandy 1999; Sheard and Power 2000; Morgan 2002). Changes in attitude regarding human waste occurred concomitant with these developments in domestic and public engineering; consequent changes in architecture and town organization combined to sharpen sensitization to body odor and the odor of body products. The conceit in *Perfume* (Suskind 1987 [1985]) – that the character Grenouille might lack olfactory discrimination between the pleasant and disgusting – is only intelligible in a society where the acts and products of elimination are managed.

Elimination is possibly the only behavior that today still has a totally dedicated space, although variations in plumbing fixtures highlight differences across cultures of inspecting and disposing of human waste. In domestic privacy, individuals may or may not routinely take note of the products of elimination and check for signs of abnormality. Cultural attitudes to the body determine what activities are exposed or performed in public and what body parts are visible, and various strategies are employed to maintain an illusion of privacy where the boundaries are confused. In public toilet stalls "usually only the toilet itself is spot-lit, the space around the fixture [is] left ill defined in semi-darkness, lest one all too easily disrupt the fantasy of privacy" (Morgan 2002:8). Only in parts of China do multiple-hole toilets continue, requiring that individuals defecate in public and ignore the intrusions of others' farts and smells, but even here, partitions between individual seats introduce a privacy not required for urination. Toilet stalls make the public private; at urinals, privacy is maintained by the etiquette that men look ahead without focus, or maintain conversation with their fellow pissers as though the waist up were disengaged from the business below. The rituals and paraphernalia of the lavatory, and in some places bidet, toilet paper and water, soap and room fresheners emphasize that defecation should be discreet and discrete. And through socialization into its practices and 'proper' language, the child learns to understand the abstractions of propriety and privacy.

The emphasis on teaching a child to master control over bowels and bladder has resonance in loss of control among those who are older. Depending on cultural context and material circumstance, an infant may simply be held out from the mother's body to defecate, or feces are captured and cleared away with a cloth, but a growing child learns to recognize feelings of fullness and pressure, and to control evacuation until finding an appropriate place. In industrialized societies, we shift from admiring regular motions as a sign of a well-fed baby and successful parenting, to the dramas, disappointments and excitement of potty-training success, to the tears of the young child who has had an 'accident,' until elimination is a matter out-of-sight, behind closed doors. Bowel and bladder control prove independence and maturity.

The internalized notion of being in control of one's own body is lost with a colostomy, an ileostomy or a urostomy. In this chapter, I focus on people who have had major surgery, either urgently as with cancer or injury, or after a period of protracted illness as is typical for those who have had irritable bowel syndrome or a related disorder. They are all people who are no longer able to eliminate or to control elimination, and so have a stoma, an opening on the side of their abdomen, for this purpose. With a urostomy, a piece of intestine, separated from the rest, is drawn through the opening and attached to the ureter to allow urine to drain. With a colostomy, the large bowel is diverted to the stoma opening; with an ileostomy the small intestine is brought to the abdomen to allow fecal material to pass. The basic appliances for a urostomy, colostomy or ileostomy are the same. A one-piece flange is adhered to the skin around the stoma, and is connected to a changeable, watertight bag that fills with urine or feces. Alternately, a person may opt for a two-piece system, with a drainable or closed-end pouch which can be removed and reapplied without removing the wafer or barrier over the stoma. Bags come in different shapes, sizes and materials. Additional products are available to reduce problems: paste to smooth scar tissue, folds and wrinkles, and ensure secure sealing; barrier film to protect skin from adhesive trauma, friction and chemical irritation from urine or fecal liquid; deodorant drops to add to a urostomy bag to reduce odor. In addition, some people with colostomies (but not ileostomies) are able to dispense with the bag. Instead, they wear a small cap over the stoma and irrigate routinely, usually every second day, introducing warm water through a funnel into the gut, then flushing the motion into the toilet bowel through an irrigation sleeve.

Stoma surgery is an end-point of a serious condition: urostomy for bladder bifida; colostomy or ileostomy, depending on the extent of the resection, for colorectal cancer or other gastrointestinal cancer, an intestinal blockage or internal injury, inflammatory bowel diseases (Crohn's disease or ulcerative colitis), or uncommonly, an intestinal abscess or congenital condition.[1] Like other conditions that I consider in this book, these are not new procedures. Hardy (1989) refers to accounts of colostomy (in the lower back) from the sixteenth and seventeenth centuries, and by the mid-nineteenth century, stoma surgery was common for bowel obstruction and rectal cancer (see Figure 4.1). Its prevalence increased and its success improved from the end of the century with developments in anesthesia and antibiotics.

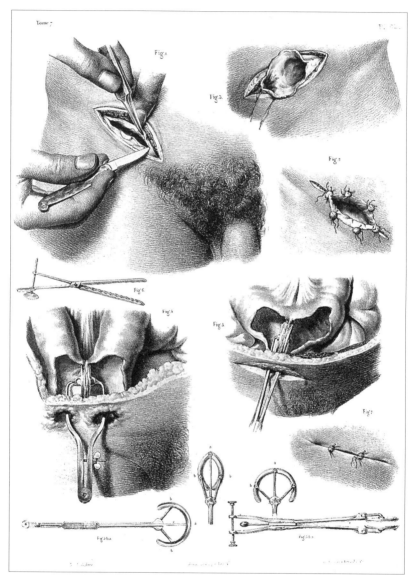

Figure 4.1 Nineteenth century stoma surgery; Wellcome Littre's inguinal colostomy. Stages in the operation; 1840.
Courtesy of Wellcome Library, London.

Sara's Story

Sara's narratives of ongoing struggles with her body highlight the quest for personal restitution and social re-integration – normality – of many whom I interviewed. Her success as a professional in human resource management belies the tragedies and continuing struggles that have marked her life and body. The account that follows is based on her story, but in its presentation here, I have fictionalized it; her story is too dramatic, too distinctive to ensure her anonymity, with or without the use of pseudonyms. A pseudonym works well enough when de-contextualized, but context can sometimes strip its effectiveness away.[2]

Sara was 37 when I met her, the second of four children of working class parents. Her mother was Australian-born and of Anglo-Celtic background, her father an immigrant whose ability to prosper economically and socially was inhibited by the lack of recognized qualifications. He was determined his children would excel in all respects, in ways that he could not. Both parents worked long hours, her father as a laborer then carpenter in the building industry; her mother undertaking domestic work while caring for her children. The family nearly disintegrated when the youngest child died of asthma while under Sara's and her older brother's care, and her mother retreated into a private world of grief. Neither Sara nor her brother had any way to deal with their own loss or sense of responsibility. Sara's father and brother fought bitterly thereafter; the brother skipped school and his grades declined; he left home as soon as he was able. Sara and her younger brother were left at home. Sara spent hours into the night studying, seeking to meet her parents' expectations and to secure her father's approval of her scholastic gains and worthiness. In turn, he denigrated her efforts, and prohibiting the recreational and personal freedom that her school friends enjoyed, pushed her harder still.

From early childhood Sara had eaten for comfort; from the age of 10 she stole and hoarded food and binged when she could escape parental surveillance: "I think I had a tremendous craving to be loved, or to feel like I was loved, and when I didn't get that, I turned to food. I can remember feeling that I was huge. I look back now at photos from that time, and I am no different from the next girl, you know." By the time she was in middle high school, she was bingeing regularly, and was very overweight, and because of this, she routinely followed binge eating with purging, taking laxatives in order to feel "really clean. I didn't think they made you lose weight. I knew they didn't make you lose weight in the long term, but I knew they made me feel clean." As she described her experience:

> I learnt very early on that I could control my feelings and my weight, and my body image, by doing that [bingeing], and even into my 20s I kept that going. I had an overwhelming feeling that I was dirty, and in order to clean myself I needed to binge. Part of the side effects of bingeing is that you get a feeling of comfort, and when I got that comfy feeling, I kind of wanted to get it out of me because it was so foreign. It was so foreign to me that it couldn't stay inside me; I didn't deserve to have that comfort feeling. You know, I only knew punishment.... I felt I wasn't good enough. I wasn't the perfect child as I think my father was seeking. I think a lot of that earlier behavior was about rejection and abandonment, and about trying to be the perfect child that my parents had wanted, and being the one who was alive, and never living up to expectations. Everything went wrong, and nothing [I did] was ever good enough.

At the same time, she imposed on herself a rigid exercise regime, running miles each day to punish herself for breaches in a diet imposed to effect control over her life. During this period, Sara felt, she said, "omnipotent. I was all-powerful and nothing could touch me. I had total control. I would like to go back, not to that size, but to that feeling, if that makes sense." From early adolescence and into adulthood, too, Sara began to cut her breasts, labia and stomach, wearing long-sleeved shirts and trousers year round to hide fresh scabs and faded scars. At 22, she was admitted to the hospital after cutting deeply into her abdomen. She was obese, and had acute stomach pain, rectal bleeding and fever. She was diagnosed with toxic megacolon, characterized by an extremely dilated colon, abdominal distension, and pain, outcomes of her frequent episodes of bingeing and purging. Warnings from the attendant doctor of the potential lethal nature of her condition, the possibility of a colostomy, and the likelihood of psychotherapy following discharge from the hospital had little impact other than to compound Sara's sense of failure. She continued to cut, binge and purge. As she explained, it was as if an external force were controlling her, "my thoughts, my feelings, my body size, how I look, what happens to me in my life, it controls that. So it is almost like a projection, and it is always negative things."

One year later, following peritonitis from a perforated colon, Sara had surgery to remove much of her colon and rectum, and to create an ileoanal reservoir ('J pouch') while leaving the anal sphincter muscle intact. But she continued to binge and purge between scheduled surgeries, leading to blockages and consequently a permanent colostomy. Her subsequent difficulty with diet caused embarrassing noise and odor. Problems along skin creases caused the flange of the colostomy bag to lift off her skin, resulting in leaks, tissue breakdown and infections, and excoriation and ulceration of the stoma. Finally, Sara developed a painful parastomal hernia that caused recurrent leakage and messier accidents both day and night. The hernia was removed and the stoma re-sited. Since then, the stoma has been re-sited three times. But still, Sara continues to fight her own sense of failure by bingeing, purging, and cutting, with rituals executed with exquisite planning:

> It's a special routine. I used to buy food and laxatives, and vomit. Then I started to use ipecac (an emetic). I learnt that from reading other peoples' tricks of the trade. I thought, oh, I will never use ipecac. I don't need to use that to throw up. And one day I lost my gag reflex. I went straight around to the pharmacy and said, my 2 year old has just drunk all this alcohol and, um, the doctor now wants me to give him impecac, and can I have some please? So now I use it all the time, and I just go to different chemists so they don't recognize me. And if I drive past a chemist, I can actually taste the ipecac, which is just revolting, oh, I can feel it now. As it is supposed to be [revolting], of course. So, I tell work I have a migraine. Then I go out to a shop – different shops in different suburbs, where people won't recognize me – and I collect all the food I think I want to eat that will make me feel good, like ice-cream and cake and so on, and I make sure that the food will be easy to vomit back up again. I am really obsessed with someone knowing, like someone coming from work to check up on me, so I draw the curtains, shut the windows, put the cat outside. I lay the food out on the floor, and then I eat off the floor. I have a thing about being so vulgar that I eat off the floor. Then I stop for lunch and eat something healthy. Once you've thrown it up, it's out, and it's like it never went in. So then it is okay to have a healthy lunch, and then I go back to bingeing and vomiting again until I am exhausted. I didn't, I never plan whole day binges. It's like, I have finished my fish and chips, I've finished my bread, I've finished my ice-cream, I have finished everything like that, what am I going to have now? After you've thrown up. Because throwing up makes you feel physically exhausted, too. And you lie on the

bathroom floor panting after you have thrown up enough. You go a bit black and dizzy. And I think vomiting is an acceptable form of being sick. If you are vomiting, you must be really sick.

To counter the abuses of diet, Sara sporadically spends long periods in a gym – one day spending fifteen hours there – in a desperate effort to reduce her weight because she believes that people will "take my intelligence more seriously if I'm a normal weight." But Sara sees her weight, and the tracks, scars and ruts across her abdomen, as constant embodied reminders of her faults. As she notes, bodywork "takes a lot of energy and a lot of thought time that could be put into other things." Now, too, cutting, bingeing and purging, intermittent exercise and erratic changes in weight are ways that Sara copes not only with feeling fat and bad, but also with having a stoma. The stoma she finds particularly repugnant:

> Dying is not as bad as living with an ileostomy. See dying, I wasn't scared of dying. Having a stoma is a constant reminder that I am bad; that I have done something to hurt myself. And I think more and more, I am realizing that this is not going to go away, that this is not just a phase. You know, I am realizing that when I am 60 or 70, if I live that long, I will still have a bag, and it is not going to go away tomorrow. An operation is not going to fix it up. It's a constant reminder of how I have treated my body. I can't take away this sign of what I have done to my body. I was so bad that this is my punishment for the rest of my life, you know.

For Sara, the stoma now is the focal object of contempt and disgust, and in consequence she is provoked to return to cutting:

> And when I get it, the feeling of obsession, it is terrible. Like now, it is focusing on the stoma. Once I cut my stoma off; I just got a pair of scissors and went chop! I thought, well I will be okay now, because it won't work and I will be normal, and I will just sew it up. I just wanted it to go back to normal; it will just go back to how it should be…. I think my body image at the moment is very flawed, and it will never be, never be how I dreamt it to be. [I would like to] have a body that could eat three meals a day and not gain or lose weight, blend in with people, and not be outside of the norm. That would be my dream body. I will never have that.

Thus Sara struggles constantly with her body and her role in making it.

Sara's constant struggles with her body are extreme. Few people I interviewed had such complex psychological backgrounds or family trauma, although the majority certainly did not live simple comfortable lives devoid of physical or psychic pain except for a single surgical event. For some, as I shall illustrate, surgery and its outcomes were traumatic; for others, stoma surgery was variously life saving, inevitable, or a relief from ongoing health problems. And while the lives of some people were punctured by surgery or its antecedents, others had experiences, positive and negative, preceding and succeeding surgery, that spilled into their illness narratives, muddying both their and my understandings of singular events.

A Rose(bud) by Any Other Name

All I was told by the stoma therapist was that they'd be creating a nice little rosebud on my stomach, which was quite amusing considering the amount of intestine that they actually made it out of. It didn't look like a rosebud to me. (Jane)

I looked at it, and it was really swollen and big, and I didn't ... they hadn't told me what to expect, because they assumed that I would know all about it and I didn't, I didn't remember it, and I just about died when I saw it, I just got a huge shock.... And since then I've had nightmares. I have this nightmare that it's turned inside out, that it's squeezed itself out the right way. I'm sure it was just the shock of them not preparing me for what I was going to see. And I was scared that it was going to come off in my hand, and what am I going to do with it now, and all that kind of stuff. (Rachel)

He made my stoma into the lovely little rosette that it is now. (Grandma Frog)

It was a common trope among men and women to refer to their stoma as a rose, a rosebud or a rosette, and a common way, too, for surgeons to prepare their patients, to soften the disquiet of the soft tissue aperture that they must use, thereafter, to remove waste manually. For some, it was a helpful metaphor, dispelling fears of offensive odor and appearance. For others the reality disproved the metaphor.

As I have suggested, stoma surgery and the resultant stoma are part of a complex biography of the body, taking on particular significance in light of other events. Few men or women narrated a story of their surgery

Figure 4.2
Abdominal
section
showing stoma
with wafer.
Courtesy of
Australia Council
of Stoma
Associations
Incorporated.

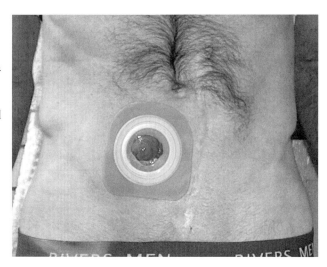

without detours into other medical, surgical and personal complications. Stoma surgery never occurred without a complex medical prehistory – it was always a final resort for treatment, as many participants reminded me, and it was often one of a number of surgeries, including multiple bladder or bowel operations, but also mastectomy and hysterectomy, other kinds of cancer, and other chronic illnesses. The history of the surgery itself, occurring for many people after extended medical treatment, influenced how people understood the stoma in relation to their sense of self and being in the world.

Maxine, for example, was 50 and with no real history of ill health at the time she saw her general practitioner for a problem with reflux. She was referred for an endoscopy and colonoscopy. The endoscopy confirmed the presence of heliobacter pylori (implicated in peptic ulcers and other digestive problems); this was successfully treated with medication. But the colonoscopy also showed some granulation. Six months later, Maxine had what she understood would be exploratory surgery. The surgery led to the diagnosis of a duodenal ulcer, Crohn's disease and a distended colon; five hours later, with three blood transfusions, Maxine had had an ileostomy. Her storytelling, not surprisingly, is marked by drama as well as pragmatism:

> I had nothing different before the operation, and now I have the ileostomy for life – unless the wonders of medicine can find something that will make a reversal 100 percent okay – but I'm not holding my

breath. The scar's about twelve inches down my middle. That doesn't worry me at all; at least I have something to put on my passport now as an identifying mark! I don't like the fact that I have a small hernia which will not get smaller and my tummy sticks out and is a bit flabby. Also because of the amount of fluid [water] that I have to drink to keep everything moving, I seem to have got flabbier in my legs, tops of arms, and around the torso. But I think the pink stoma is quite cute – it does look like a rosebud – it doesn't really worry me at all. It is something I have to live with, and I can cope with it. While I know that the current bag system I use [a very low profile two piece] is far more advanced than the old rubber bags I've heard people talking about, I wish there was something a bit less medical looking. You often find that the producers of stomal supplies do not have a stoma and can't really understand our concerns.

Maxine "keeps a close watch" on her stoma to make sure "it is healthy at all times, especially the skin area where the flanges attach," because, as she understands it, irritations and reactions can easily occur, causing further discomfort. Her pragmatism reflects her sense of choice: "body image versus being alive."

Other people had even more complicated and protracted medical histories and stories of surgeries. Colleen, for example, was 58 at the time of her storytelling. She had had a total hysterectomy for chronic endometriosis at the age of 30, but she continued to experience severe pelvic pain. At the age of 52, she was diagnosed with bowel cancer and given a colostomy. Twelve months later, following a major obstruction of the colon, the colostomy was converted to an ileostomy. Subsequently, a tumor blocked both her right and left ureter, and her left kidney ceased to function. Several months later, she began to bleed from her bladder, and she had surgery to cauterize a number of veins. The anesthetic spinal block administered for this surgery led to permanent anesthesia of her lower pelvic area, and, probably due to surgery, first one, then a second, fistula. Seven weeks later, weighing 42 kilos (92 pounds), she left the hospital dually incontinent. Her right kidney began to fail two years later, and she now uses a nephrostomy bag that she explains "plays a vital part of keeping [me] alive." She has, she says, always been concerned more with cleanliness than beauty for positive acceptance. Now, her life is dominated by managing the stoma. Like Sara, she, too, struggles to make sense of all this and to find an identity outside of her poor health:

Of all that has happened to me [incontinence] has been the hardest
thing to bear. I cannot adequately describe the indignity of it and the
limiting effect it has had on my already restricted lifestyle. I have two
bags, a spinal block, dual incontinence, wasted muscles, gaunt face,
and scrawny neck and arms. Of all of these, however, it is the incontinence that has destroyed my confidence. I am tied to the toilet for
hours on end. Since the incontinence has become part of my daily
existence I've been restricted to dark colors with patterns to try to disguise my frequent 'accidents.' I struggle to find a meaning in living
with a disease that so impairs my self-esteem. I always coped by freezing the feelings and avoiding the issue. Now, I just feel numb and very
tired, I don't see myself as a whole person anymore.

Unlike Colleen and Sara, Adrienne's health problems occurred over a
shorter period of twelve years, from the time her children were adolescents
and she was in her early 40s. After two years of increasingly heavy periods
and painful intercourse, she sought medical attention and was admitted to
the hospital for a routine laparoscopy. Recovery was unproblematic, but
she was sore and bloated. Seventeen hours later, she had still not voided
and so was catheterized. Fifteen hours later again, when she had failed to
void again, the catheter was re-inserted and left in situ for "two to three
days." After she had experienced urethral spasms, she was given a suprapubic catheter and bladder retraining, and after five weeks, she was taught
to self-catheterize. Two years on, still with incontinence, heavy periods
and painful intercourse, she was admitted for a second laparoscopy and
cystoscopy to examine the interior of the bladder. This was followed by
the insertion of a large bore suprapubic catheter to allow for adequate
drainage, more self-catheterization, and psychological assessment (she
was found "very sane"). A year later, she agreed to surgical re-siting of
the ureter with bladder flap surgery, so that she could catheterize without
pain while the ulcers in her urethra, due to extended self-catheterization,
healed. This surgery was repeated twice. Four years later, she had an ileal
diversion, and was readmitted to the hospital twice for bowel obstruction,
and subsequently, after continuing pain and infection, her bladder was
removed and she was given a urostomy. Since then she has been hospi-
talized on multiple occasions for urostomy repair, bowel obstruction, and
hysterectomy. In describing this saga of surgeries, she is intermittently
angry and depressed.

In contrast, Gertrude's story of chronic illness and surgery is braided with optimism. Her health problems began around fifteen years before we met, when she began to experience constipation and blood spotting. She was advised to change her diet. The problems continued, however, and after three years, she was diagnosed first with ulcerative colitis, then with Crohn's disease. She was given sulfur drugs, and when her health deteriorated, steroids. Her weight ballooned. Her husband became "very stand-offish," withdrawing from her sexually and making hurtful comments about her weight. She continued to suffer from sporadic diarrhea and constipation for ten years, at which time a fistula that had tracked alongside her vagina presented through her labia. Her health deteriorated rapidly, and she was admitted to the hospital with excruciating pain from the labial fistula, an intestinal abscess, and an abscess on the side of her anus. A second recto-vaginal fistula developed while she was an inpatient. In two weeks, she had four operations on various abscesses and fistulas; she looked, she said, "like a torture chamber down there with all these drains and everything." She was still constipated and febrile. Five weeks later, she was given a colostomy. She described this as the best thing that had happened to her: she feels she can finally "live again." Like Maxine, therefore, Gertrude's pragmatism and acceptance of the procedure, the stoma, and the need to manage it to prevent excoriation and to minimize accidents, derive from her sense of balance and her understanding of stoma surgery as a measure of last resort.

The Moral Responsibility for Illness

Public health education and health promotion messages increasingly emphasize the importance of reporting abnormal body signs to ensure early diagnosis, hence preventing severe morbidity or avoidable mortality. The 'public' is warned that signs of change to the surface or the felt experience of the body are (or can be) signs of illness. A mole that darkens might be melanoma; a lump in the breast, cancer; a pain in the chest, heart disease. We are implored, in any public health campaign, to improve health outcomes through early intervention, to know our own bodies and to report changes (to medical authorities). For this purpose, the body is separate from 'self' – it is an object for monitoring, surveillance and control. For people with digestive and gastrointestinal problems, the toilet bowl is the surveillance site for evidence of pathology – the presence of mucus or blood, unusual consistency or color, offensive odor. Such signs of dysfunction, including bodily changes that might once have been ignored or sloughed off, are gathered together by the doctors to whom men and women present as symptoms of pathology, clustered as potentially related, and translated algorithmically into syndromes that require further investigation and treatment. Yet the health problems of people who end up with stomas are so ordinary – urinary frequency, constipation or diarrhea –that there remains a suspicion in the public imaginary, if not in medicine, that the conditions are invented, the sufferers malingerers, diagnosticians opportunists. People with conditions such as ulcerative colitis and Crohn's disease, for example, like those with urinary incontinence or chronic pelvic pain, are typically reticent of their health problems to avoid accusations of 'imagined' illness. Days off work for chronic conditions are typically represented – in the media, in workplace accident and occupational health enquiries, and in statements of personal opinion – as evidence of turpitude or laxity. This is not only in the imagination of participants; one woman I interviewed was reminded publicly, on her retirement, that her workplace had 'carried her' for years.

Individual responsibility is insinuated in illness trajectories, the breaches of the body assumed to reflect the social person. This is a real tension for people with embattled or ambiguous bodies, including those who have to manage their body as an object, as occurs in caring for a stoma to prevent abrasions, lesions and infection, in changing bags, and so on. The tension exists because the body has to be managed; in terms of self-image and in terms of social relationships, each person needs to separate the self and the physical body – the 'real' you from the body-with-stoma, the object – related to *who you are* and *who others assume you to be*. Thus Rachel reflected on the way the denial of her stoma, and on the congenital abnormalities that contributed to this and other surgery, impacted upon her as a young woman:

> I mean the psychology of the time was that you had to normalize us, you know, just pretend that it wasn't there, and that's what I think they [parents] did. I think it was pretty much, you know, an okay way to handle it, but I also think that it was affecting their psychological make-up because then they could ignore it and pretend that they had a normal kid, because I never … nobody was actually nice to me about it, because you've got to pretend, you've got to treat her as normal, no different from other kids. And so there was never actually any "Oh,

you poor thing" or "You've got to go to hospital." There was none of that actually loving stuff; I think that they just felt they had to do it, you know, it was embarrassing, they had this kid that wasn't normal.

Most people struggled against ideas of causality that linked their physical and psychological health, yet also explained their health problems in relation to their own prior actions. As described above, for example, Sara saw her stoma as proof of her own failings, embodied, too, in the cycles of bingeing, purging and cutting. Popular notions of causation influenced how people with cancer responded to the diagnosis and were regarded by others, and illness was often represented as self-inflicted or warranted; people felt that the disease was due to personal failure to 'eat properly' or control their weight. Rhonda had had bowel cancer and a colostomy, then breast cancer and a mastectomy:

> Maybe I'm just a person who's a bit self-pitying. I know some people who can go through breast cancer, and say, oh well, that's that, end of story. But I took it very personally somehow and thought it wasn't fair. The first time round [when treated for bowel cancer], I said to the doctors, "Has this been caused by stress? Because I've been a widow and I've had a hard life. And my first husband needed nursing." And [the doctor] said, "No, no, nothing to do with stress. If you ate more corn like the people in Africa, you'd never have had bowel cancer." I think now some doctors recognize that there is such a thing as stress and they even talk about it. But at the time it was all because I hadn't eaten enough vegetables and I'd probably eaten too much meat … and I thought that this sort of horrendous problem (a stoma) should not happen to nice people. So I must be a nasty person for it to happen to me. But you do try to question why. There may be no answers and you think, if I'd played more sport, if I'd eaten less butter, if I'd … whatever.

Rhonda tried to conceptualize her illness in a way that was empowering:

> I suppose for a lot of my life I've had that feeling that I'm not really very worthwhile. But I think if I look at it objectively, the problems I've had medically may have made me more confident. I used to worry about what people thought about me, and I wondered if they thought I was a worthwhile sort of person or not. I think having had to face these problems, I'm less concerned about what people think of me and I've probably got more internal resources. I'm not so concerned about what others think. So that's quite a big shift for a person, I suppose.

A number of people like Rhonda subscribed to multiple causes of their poor health – the stresses of everyday life and diet, for instance. Personal etiologies enabled them to make biographic sense of their illness and surgery. Roger attributed his colorectal cancer to stress, "definitely way up on the top and diet very close behind." He also blamed his former wife, and reflected on his own role in the stress that led to his stoma: "If I get angry, it's at me because I did the wrong thing. I married the wrong woman." Like Sara, therefore, several people saw the stoma as evidence of their reprehensibility; their past incapacity and poor judgment were now sutured into their bodies.

The Body Exposed

In her famous Public Cervix Announcement (Kapsalis 1997), Annie Sprinkle exposed her cervix to anyone who wished to view it, but in order for her cervix to be seen, she also displayed other body parts almost always hidden from view – her vulva, anus, vagina. Her name, employing a euphemism for urinating, alone breached public/private boundaries of politeness. Not everyone has seen their own genitals. They don't after surgery:

> One of the things that came to my mind, when I was thinking of your visit and this discussion, was with regard to the surgery and the scarring. In thirteen years, I've never looked at those scars. I just couldn't bring myself to do it. I suppose it's a private part of your body, but it was a major trauma of course to know that you would have no rectum, that every muscle is taken, that you would have a stoma. (Betty)

For people with rectal or bowel cancer, feces stained with blood and mucus may be the first sign of danger, and the anus and the processes of evacuation take on sudden importance. Blood in urine, too, is an immediate indication of pathology, but so may be the frequent need to go to the toilet, or the inability to pass water or stool, or the lack of control over bladder or bowel. In all cases, these abnormalities, often accompanied by pain, eventually overwhelm embarrassment, lack of familiarity and the reluctance of being exposed, and lead to a medical consultation. People spoke recurrently of the loss of dignity and the embarrassment associated with incontinence, but in the face of serious illness, they emphasized that the indignity and discomfort of the physical examination, the pain of surgery, and for those with rectal cancer, the clumsiness of lying bottom-up for radiotherapy, faded. Phoenix recalled his embarrassment when he finally presented to his general practitioner with blood in feces: "He (the doctor) threw me up on the couch, got out the rubber glove, said something along the lines of 'please relax.' I've tried to keep people away from that area for a lot of my life, so relaxing was not easy, but anyway he did the examination."

Urinary 'plumbing problems' are normalized for women since they are constructed largely as outcomes of childbearing and aging. Consequently, there is some space for women to talk about difficulties associated with continence and constipation. However, women must necessarily now touch as well as talk about their bodies. Adrienne, for instance, had had ongoing problems emptying her bladder, and had to learn to self-catheterize: "And, as if all that had already happened was not already degrading and embarrassing enough, I now had to endure this bloody therapist lying at the other end of the bed peering at my fanny and telling me where to aim. The only light-hearted relief was from a friend who said, 'Just go for the third hole from the back of the neck.'"

Like urinary incontinence, for women hemorrhoids are normalized as the result of childbirth. Men lack these excuses of embodied history to explain away such problems. Other signs of anal and urethral ill health – fissures, itching, discharge, swelling – are as embarrassing as they are uncomfortable, implying poor personal hygiene and inadequate body maintenance. The anti-pruritic cream Anusol, by its very name, advertises the condition to others at the supermarket check-out and causes as much embarrassment to consumers as does the purchase of incontinence pads, although in Australia the increasing frequency of advertisements of incontinence pads, like menstrual pads and tampons twenty years earlier, suggests that such boundaries of discretion are being eroded with the prevalence of the conditions.

The anus and urethral opening are body parts rarely exposed, the butt of jokes that attest to their taboo nature. The taboo pertains not only when individuals must clean the bodies and handle the waste of others, as occurs in caregiving (Isaksen 2002), but also with respect to their own bodies. Both before and after surgery, the association of health problems with dirtiness is emphasized in the techniques of diagnosis and surgery via the steps with which individuals must engage through manual bowel prep in order to be 'clean' for surgery: twenty-four hours on a clear liquid diet, the unpleasant ingestion of barium meal or a similar laxative, sometimes also an enema. Closing the urethra or anus, and locating a stoma on the abdomen to enable the manual removal of the products of the bladder or bowel, give further visibility and vocality to body parts and functions, bringing literally and metaphorically to the fore that previously hidden between the legs and at the back of the body. Sometimes the memory stays. Perdita talked about phantom farts: "You know if anyone expels wind from their anus it gets out, it's gone, you have that dilation of the rectum. I mean I sometimes get phantom feelings there. It soon goes, but it is like a phantom." And Betty reflects:

> The extraordinary thing is that I can still remember the sort of bearing down feeling of needing to go to the toilet, of needing to pass feces. Of course all those nerves and everything have been taken away, but the body still says you've got waste products in there that need to get out and I sometimes lose track of which day I have to do it. The day you don't have to do it is very pleasant because you think, good, I don't have to worry about this today. And then the next day you sort of think, oh yes, I'm starting to feel a bit uncomfortable, of course, I've got to irrigate tonight, or whatever.

As already noted, the stoma requires constant care, demanding far greater self-consciousness than a wipe without looking, a blot, or a shake. The body can no longer be managed by itself:

> At first it was yuck, yuck, poo. Oh, I have got a bit on my fingers, oh quick, wash it off. Now, I don't worry or panic about. (Gertrude)

> I was in hospital for three weeks and I think I had a fair bit of morphine for this surgery, it was pretty drastic, and of course I decided that I wouldn't eat, see, because if I didn't eat I wouldn't make any mess, because the thought of having feces coming from the front of your body....Well, I remember that I'd heard vaguely that people with that sort of condition had a bag and I thought, to walk around for the rest of my life with a bag that was going slop, slop was not going to be very pleasant at all. So it was a very primitive way of trying to cope with it, by thinking if I don't eat, then I won't have to deal with the feces. But it was pretty drastic. But I did know that I had a son who was 14 and if possible, I had to pull through to look after him. So I think the desire to live was very strong. (Rhonda)

Learning to look after a stoma, as well as to undergo radiotherapy after surgery, reinforced the indignity that some people felt when they first walked into a clinic:

I really don't like anyone else sort of touching my stoma at all. It's my job and I don't fancy the stoma therapy nurse coming around and changing it because I suppose it's got something to do with indignity. No one else has people, you know, running around their bums and changing dirty nappies, so why should they do it for me. (Jane)

For people with cancer, the clinic provides a sanitary space in which vulnerability to disease overrides perceived insults to dignity; the primary task at hand is to control cancer. As Perdita describes it, patients are medicalized and their body parts fragmented, their 'selves' secondary to the site of disease and its status as the focal point of radiotherapy for adjuvant treatment. The stoma and its care slide into the backwash; the task of learning to handle this new body part and its products is sidelined.

Space and Place

While the intestinal waste that extrudes into a stoma bag is unfamiliar, we all handle body products at various times. Menstrual blood, sweat, saliva, tears, and mucus flow regardless, by and large, and need to be managed. The more innocuous the product, the lesser the need to remove it hastily and discreetly, but even tears out of place or context – at the wrong moment, the wrong time – are problematic. Other products, viscous, colored, odorous, are more problematic, and need to be absorbed or quickly wiped away (Douglas 1966). Sanitary pads and tampons, antiperspirants and handkerchiefs are simple technologies that allow us to minimize border transgressions of the body and sanitize individual bodies in social contexts. Mouthwash prevents halitosis from fouling shared space. Public vomiting is clear evidence of loss of bodily (and self) control either through sudden sickness or drunkenness, the latter state itself the invasion of an out-of-control body in public space. Nail clipping, shaving, dental flossing and wound care are largely private (or semi-private – as occurs in medical clinics) activities. The primary exceptions, largely confined to purpose-specific environments, are hair-cutting and nail care. Technology allows for even greater discretion and less risk of infringement of public space: tampons collect blood internally; laser removal of body hair reduces stubble; paper tissues obviate washing mucus from cloth handkerchiefs; insulin pens allow people with diabetes to inject unobtrusively even in public. The issue is esthetic and cultural, even if wrapped in the rhetoric of infection control and 'hygiene' (again, see Douglas 1966).

Given this broad cultural emphasis on privacy and cleanliness, men and women with fecal or urinary incontinence internalized notions of themselves as willful, lacking physical and social control, and as vulnerable to public disclosure. Incontinence stripped them of social membership through constraints on their mobility, and stripped them, too, symbolically, of gender and sexuality. As one woman explained, incontinence and the necessary management of the body "make you feel not the woman you were."[3] Pre-surgery, those who had chronic inflammatory disease and incontinence organized their lives around toilet facilities and the prevention of accidents. Vanessa recalled that "the worst part of my life was always needing to know where a toilet was whenever I left the house, always running to try to 'make' it." People spoke of endless hours sitting on toilets attempting to defecate, in agony with constipation or with urinary tract infections; routinely shuffling from doctor's clinic to hospital for cystoscopies and colonoscopies; being recommended to counselors and psychologists for assessment for conditions presumed imaginary; experimenting with diet, herbs, naturopathic treatments, acupuncture, relaxation; and agreeing to temporary stomas and self-catheterizing. These multiple strategies would continue to the point when many, exhausted, agreed to a permanent stoma. Until this time, their lives were dictated by incontinence, incapacity, embarrassment and pain.

Following surgery, with the assistance of a stoma therapy nurse, men and women with chronic disease, and those who had urgent surgery for bladder or colorectal cancer, had to learn to manage the stoma: how to attach a pouch, how and when to remove and empty it, how to clean and care for the stoma and surrounding skin, and so on. But they also had to learn to live with it comfortably, that is, to learn to be among other people without self-consciousness. People constantly negotiated their bodies to prevent accidental bumps or touch, allowing extra space around their bodies for this purpose. In Leder's terms (1990:179), they treated the site of the stoma as a thematically central tool for bodily orientation. People who had stomas manipulated their bodies when with partners; they arranged garments so that the outline of a bag could not be seen; they were vigilant of noise or odor. In interviews, they frequently sat with a hand over the stoma bag, unconsciously monitoring and guarding it while we spoke. For intimates, this surveillance reminded both of bodily change. Mia, who at the time of the interview had a temporary stoma for Crohn's disease, reflected on how this affected everyday activities:

My social life has changed dramatically since I got the ileostomy. I hate having a stoma, I hate just about everything associated with it. Like, I won't take a bath. I won't swim, mainly because I can't find anything to wear. I think if I had, you know, something that covered it properly, then I would; I haven't been swimming in over two years now and I really miss it. But your average swimsuit is very revealing. You'd be able to see the outline of the bag underneath, especially if it filled up a little bit. And I would be really embarrassed in the changing rooms and things like that. I see girls wearing hipsters, or something like that. I'd like to wear those, or a tight or swingy skirt or something like that. I mean, part of feeling sexy, I think, is feeling sexy in what you wear. And when you're wearing big baggy pants, it doesn't make you feel sexy in your own mind. And I don't like being in crowds. I don't know if I'm worried about having an accident or whether I'm worried about people brushing up against me, feeling it. It's not the stoma itself, it's actually the fact that you're emptying your bowel contents into a bag. It's the fact that I shit in a bag. And I carry it around with me all the time. There's so many things. I don't feel normal. I feel like I'm flawed and inadequate. I certainly don't feel sexy at all, you know. Not at all. I just … I don't know.

Adrienne, who had a urostomy, also spoke of her self-consciousness in public space:

I feel like a fugitive when trying on clothes in shops as helpful assistants bring stuff to the change rooms. Some days I shower three or four times a day because I don't feel clean and constantly think I can smell myself so I assume others can as well.

Despite the choices available, people often experienced difficulty finding a comfortable flange and bag, dealing with gas and odor, preventing leakage, keeping clean, protecting the peristomal skin from the stool and trauma, avoiding excoriation, and preventing damage to the stoma itself. Skin care is largely a private concern, but smell and sound are invasive; both functions and senses are out of control. Touch can be avoided or limited, one can look away or close one's eyes, but smell and sound can neither be turned off nor shut down. The body intrudes as it produces. Even ordinary breaches of the gut, tummy rumbles and farts are embarrassing, inappropriate displays of a lack of bodily control that draw attention to body functions. The owner of the indiscretion can usually walk away, disassociated, leaving a malodorous ghost of self behind. The potential sensory incursions into others' lives with a stoma, via leaks, smells and sounds, heighten the possibility of disclosure and make it difficult for people to feel 'normal' in everyday interactive contexts. As Jane explained, "I suppose it's kind of obsessive, like the main focus of my life, and it worries me that it's my main focus because, you know, who in their right mind focuses on going to the toilet? It affects me more than I'd like it to."

Hence people with stomas pay considerable attention to managing risk, and those sensitive to foods (such as cabbage and beans) that cause increased gas or odor were as concerned with input as output. Dimity, for example, took an enzyme preparation to reduce gas. Phoenix used a bag with a charcoal filter, which prevented odor although not the sound of gas escaping into the pouch. Flanges lift with perspiration in hot weather, causing odor to escape and feces or urine to leak. "You should hear us," Perdita said, "it's like the Sydney Symphony Orchestra at our conferences, because everyone's sitting around the table and you'll hear ten or fifteen different noises. We all know where it's coming from but we've all got different noises." Conferences of consumer associations and stoma therapists inevitably include substantial display areas for companies producing stoma products, all claiming to address these ubiquitous problems. For those who irrigate, the plug inserted into the stoma absorbs gas; it is removed when it has expanded, and prevents "great burping noises that can be very embarrassing, as if you're passing wind from the front of your stomach" (Betty, participant). With the exception of those who use plugs, people with a stoma have no real control: the bag fills regardless. Emptying the bag in public settings was problematic, and privacy was a 'big issue':

> You know, people in places like public toilets are always looking under the toilet door, and you know, just coming in. And then there's the odor as well and things like that. I don't worry about my odor when I'm pulling up my clothes. It's just when I'm emptying the bag and things like that. (Mia)

Men found changing bags in public places particularly problematic, as Phoenix explained:

> If I have to walk a few hundred yards or something, start to perspire, and I've had a plate on for twenty-four hours or longer, the glue breaks down with perspiration, blah, blah, blah. I can feel it coming off, you do running repairs, you know, it's embarrassing. If you go into a public toilet, whatever, what do you do then? You've got to look in the mirror

to see the thing for hygiene purposes, but I'm obese, that's what the nurse said, so the skin that's underneath never sees the light of day. If you have to do it blind, it's very, very difficult. If you use a closed bag, how are you going to empty it? You go to the toilet, put it in there, wash it out. Now what do you wash it out in, the basin? Flush the toilet, get it under there, now it's wet. If you put it back on wet, you've now got a wet patch on your shirt, whatever, it's totally impractical. So I use a closed bag system. You've got to take one bag off, and put one on. You can't see because there's no mirror there, although I carry one with me. Male toilets, there's not even a tidy bin to put rubbish in. Women's toilets, at least they have tampon bins or something similar. What I do is put them (used bags) in a receptacle outside and dispose of them the way everybody does nappies these days. I mean, put it in the garbage, what else can you do?

Dealing with these embarrassing intrusions, locating toilets, dealing with the practicalities in cases of 'accident' discourage people from spending time away from the security of their own home. Women found such accidents profoundly distressing; men tended to deal with them with bravura. Nick, for instance, appeared rather cavalier about his urostomy:

I probably drink too much, you know, with the associated problems of the odd waterbed effect. I'm always conscious of it and how it feels and, you know, "Where am I going to need to change it today, tomorrow, the day after?" I've probably let it go a little longer at times out of laziness. As long as it's not, you know, hanging off and stinking, I don't care. If I go swimming I'll leave my shirt on, et cetera, because the last thing I need is a bloody eight-year-old kid coming up going, "What's that?" You avoid the stares and whispers.

Phoenix also had accidents after heavy drinking:

I've had bad accidents like, not long after I had the operation, I got severely in my cups [drunk] one evening and the bag had fallen off and I didn't even know 'cause I was so out of it, which was pretty dreadful. I excreted all over everything, all the doorknobs, in the bathroom and I was totally unaware of it until the kids told me the next morning. They were weird, the sheer embarrassment of it…

Many, though, have accidents – leaks or a burst bag – without warning, and unrelated to breaches in diet or drinking. Losing control is to lose independence, and to be seen to do so in public, as occurs with 'accidents' of the bowel or bladder, is profoundly humiliating. People who find it difficult to predict their need for the use of a toilet manipulate public space and map the environment so that they are never too far in the case of an emergency; so important is this that the Australian government produces a national public toilet map. And still emergencies and accidents happen, with accompanying embarrassment and distress. Perdita described one such incident at length:

> I was in a shopping centre, and I had to change bags. And I slipped. I was changing in a public toilet and there was water on the floor. My shoe went from under me just as I was taking the bag off, and I lost my balance and I fell this way, and the bag with the feces went all down the front of my trousers. I burst into tears. And there is no paper in the toilets now, there's only hand dryers, so I am trying to clean it off my jeans with toilet paper. I was horrified, but I also thought, I've got to get to work now and clean myself up, and get constructive and do all these things that have to be done and get it out of the way. So I held my bag in front of me and headed for a clothes shop. But I was so aware of the odor, you have no idea, it was just awful. I mean people understand if there is a child around and they have dirty pants or a dirty nappy, but when an adult … I mean they sort of step back about ten feet, and I felt everybody was stepping back from me. When I went into the shop, I briefly explained what had happened and said "I need to buy a pair of pants and I would like an extra plastic bag so I can wrap up these ones." And the girl was lovely; she went to a lot of trouble to make sure I was well screened, away from people, not only because of the odor. But then there was the embarrassment like you wouldn't believe, and that made me really angry. You never, ever, ever get used to the fact that this happens. I hope that as I get older I am still in control of it, because if ever the day comes that I am not, I would rather be dead.

In private spaces, too, boundaries overflow in persistent distressing ways. Stained underwear and damp and odorous bed sheets are reminders of the body that overflows, contaminating one's bed partner and oneself, leaving the individual vulnerable, under a shower while his or her partner strips and remakes the bed. Such chaotic leaks are the surface signs of illnesses that, complicated by pain, weight loss and lethargy, make miserable the lives of those so afflicted. For many, chemotherapy and other kinds of surgery have limited effectiveness, and stoma surgery, temporary or permanent, can be a 'turning of the corner,' the beginning of a 'new life.' But stoma surgery for people with either chronic or acute disease is feared as much as welcomed, with relief from symptoms or reduction of risk of early death weighed against the challenges of now having to manage elimination as a manual not a natural activity.

As indicated above, self-consciousness of having a stoma bag, of the need to empty it in public and the possibility of accidents, made many men and women reluctant to leave the safe environments of their own homes. Daryl's experience was extreme. He began to work with a therapist to overcome his anxiety about the bag and the consequent agoraphobia:

> The therapist told me how to cope with things and I tried doing what he suggested; some of the things worked, some didn't work. Gradually, I sort of was able to cope with it, a long process, say five years before I felt confident and competent. I remember the first time at work, when I went back, sitting there with the bag and worrying about noises and smells. Gradually I forced myself to go to things, like football or concerts or the races. It took quite awhile just to sit among people and not worry. There was one thing that was a big setback. I caught the train to work, it's quite a long trip, and I started using public transport a lot because that's what the therapist suggested I do. So I'd put a bag on in the morning and fix it up again when I got to work. Several times I'd walk to the train and I'd have to turn around and go home, change the bag and try again. But the thing about the major setback was, on the train, I heard one teenage boy say to his friend, "he's the one that smells." And that was the worst. Because you can't smell yourself, you're not sure, you're doing the best you can. It destroyed the whole urge to even try to get out and about.

Daryl was not alone. While most people developed various coping strategies to minimize inconvenience and embarrassment, a number experienced little improvement in quality of life and several were depressed:

> More and more I have little interest in going out. Do I allow myself to become a recluse or do I make the effort to fill as 'normal' a role as possible – to want to relate to other people in a way that is mutually energizing? I suppose I have to believe that I have still got something worthwhile to achieve even though I have lost my role and identity in the workforce. (Colleen)

Intimacy

As Isaksen (2002) illustrates in relation to the provision of care, body care and the management of incontinence stress, the boundaries that conventionally exist between kin and intimate partners are challenged with stomas. I have suggested that controlling functions of the body is an integral part of socialization from infant to adult, and so is regarded as a precondition of adulthood. The illnesses that lead to surgery, and the lived experience of having a stoma, threaten fundamentally this sense of self. Husbands and wives played major roles in reaffirming the adult status of their partners post-surgery, and many participants spoke at length of the ability of their spouse or lover to accept them and their bodies after surgery. A few stayed with partners after surgery but ceased sexual relations, reinforcing their partners' fears of their loss of adulthood as well as, most immediately, their physical desirability. Sara's husband was one. While by her account he was caring, loving and supportive, they had not had sexual relations for ten years, and Sara frequently turned to this as she worried about her weight, her obsessiveness, her self-harm, and especially the presence of her stoma.

The assault on body image during extended periods of erratic diarrhea and constipation, for those with inflammatory bowel disease, and the erosion of dignity at the time of diagnosis and surgery, eat away at self-esteem and body image. This often continued after surgery. Numerous people referred to their stomachs as 'war zones,' criss-crossed with scars from the initial surgery, later operations to re-site the stomas, and scars from excoriated tissue and hernias. While women made jokes about being 'bag ladies,' most were extremely self-conscious:

> Even to this day [ten years after surgery], I still can't walk around with nothing on. It sounds ridiculous, I suppose, when you are in a relationship, but I have always used a towel or something. It [my stomach] looks like a war zone, and as you get older things start to droop down anyway, fat and loose skin, horrible, dreadful, it shouldn't be allowed to happen. It is a funny thing when I have had the bag off, and I have just put my hand there and I have actually looked in the mirror, and I have felt totally different. Totally different, just because it is not there. I just put my hand over the bit thing [stoma] and then I see a normal body. I see somebody that is normal and not disfigured. Hasn't got this thing hanging there, that I would just like to rip off and throw

away, you know, if I could. It is all to do with body image, isn't it? How does one overcome this? (Bubbaloo)

Re-establishing the sexual self was an important theme for women and men in their narratives of accommodation to surgery, whether in terms of an existing partnership or, for those not involved in a relationship at the time of surgery, their subsequent desire and ability to establish a sexual relationship (Manderson 2005). For some participants, self-consciousness was over-ridden by desire and comfortableness with their own and their partner's body, and acceptance that the surgery "made no difference" to their partner. Rhonda reflected that although she felt "mutilated," her husband wasn't "repulsed" by her body, and she felt desirous, and so they were able to resume sexual relations and to have "satisfactory sex." Other women were willing partners, provided that the surgical site, the bag and the stoma were not touched. This was the combined result of their own sense of esthetics, not wanting to remind their partner of their disfigurement, and avoiding being reminded themselves of the bag in ways that were invasive and distracting in intimacy. Others had difficulties in resuming and maintaining sexual relations with partners because of loss of libido, and they associated this with their own self-consciousness. Dimity, however, suggested that the decline of libido also had a physiological basis:

> A lot of it, sure, is body image, but when you have so much wrong with you and you are in constant pain and what not, I mean I know how I feel and I have actually got a life and a lot of these ladies don't. Most of them are under [consulting] psychiatrists a lot of the time and on anti-depressants as well as all the other crap that they are on and then there is the issue of not having children. A lot of them have tried carrying [becoming pregnant] and it has been completely unsuccessful, some just don't fall pregnant, and yeah …

Yet as she reflects on her own sexual life, Dimity returns to themes of embarrassment in relation to incontinence as well as libidinal loss:

> I remember when we first went to bed, I used to have to hang on, I was literally clenched in fear, like I never knew if I was going to be letting off wind or something more than that and it took me a long, long time to feel comfortable. Allan says, "I am not going to abandon her. She's still Dimity. She still has the same heart, she is still herself, she just doesn't have a bum that works, she doesn't have a pancreas that works – she's just fucked really." He has just been marvelous. Sometimes I

just say to him to leave me alone but I have been very conscious of this. He says he doesn't even notice the bag and everything else, but I can feel it and I know it is there. I mean there is no desire, no nothing there, and there hasn't been probably for two years. I have to force myself. And when we do have intercourse, it can just stir things up and I have never been one to cope with bad smells and I will actually vomit. I will just say, "Get off, I'm going to be sick."

For some participants, surgery foreshadowed the end of a relationship that perhaps had already been in trouble. Ross and his wife divorced because she couldn't cope with his stoma; after he had surgery, she withdrew from him sexually and emotionally. Gertrude's husband said he was not turned off by the stoma, but he withdrew sexually anyway. As already described, her history of illness included painful fistulas and abscesses running from her rectum to her labia, and she needed surgery to drain these prior to having her colon removed:

I had freaked out at the beginning because the doctor had said to me, "Well it looks like you are going to have a bag, either temporary or full-time," and I burst into tears when he first told me that, because my husband is sort of, with his record of ignoring me when I was fat and giving me a hard time, I was really worried about what it was going to be like with a bag and getting total rejection. I told him this. In turn, he reassured me that he believed in our marriage vows "through sickness and health" and they were very strong with him and that he wouldn't reject me, and that he loved me and I would still be me even if I had a bag, and I said "Fine." That was all I needed, just to hear that he wasn't going to reject me.

Sexual relations did not resume, however, and Gertrude's husband again complained that she was "too fat" for him to find her desirable. She reflected that the stoma helped her to realize that the problem was her husband's not hers, and that divorce was an option because, she said, "I do miss the physical side of life. I need to heal first but I do get frustrated … I find hankies under the bed every now and then [evidence of masturbation], so I know it [his penis] is working."

In contrast, Phoenix married his partner after surgery. He and his wife did not have intercourse for the first eighteen months of marriage, and he experienced continuing difficulties with pain on intercourse and had difficulty ejaculating. This he understood to be as a result of "the way they put the nerve endings back together." Phoenix explained that his wife was "not into body image," but he spoke of the disconcerting sound of the bag slapping against flesh during intercourse, and of his self-image:

> The other thing about self-image is the funny sex one. The best they've come up with is to wear a cummerbund [over the stoma]. Now about the only time I've ever worn a cummerbund was way back when I was doing ballroom dancing, and a more ridiculous piece of equipment I've ever come across. I mean, what's wrong with a belt? But prancing into bed with a cummerbund, I'd just feel like a bloody Christmas present or something. You're trying to hide this thing, but what do you do, draw attention to it with a bloody cummerbund!

Avoiding the post-surgical body in intimate moments was difficult, of course. Both men and women were often mortified by the sound of urine slopping in a bag (for urostomates) or the vinyl of a stoma bag slapping against the stomach of their partner, and fear that the bag might burst. Their embarrassment was far greater when this did happen, and they and their partner had to clean up feces or urine instead of completing love-making. Close partners managed leaks pragmatically, however: "Martin doesn't care at all. He just says, 'Okay, let's change the sheets. You go and hop in the shower and I'll wash the clothes'" (Fiona).

The body is a medium: our bodies act as vehicles of expression of thoughts, ideas and emotions (Grosz 1994). Bodies also act as a reflection of the self, without the conscious use of the body for this purpose, and this makes sense of people's claims of being 'normal.' Normalness captures a state of mind rather than body. As I have argued, people are neither cognizant of nor able to view their bodies in entirety; they are unable to sense their bodies' central workings, and these are taken for granted when there are no sensory or visible signs of dysfunction.[4] People therefore imagine rather than feel or view their bodies in totality, comparing the imagined body with cultural representations and stated values of normal, ideal and desirable bodies. Yet despite the imperceptibility of the body as a whole, it is still regarded literally and symbolically as a reflection of self. People are self-consciousness of their own bodies and prejudge others on the basis of their corporeality and representation. This explains why stigma attaches to bodies that are visually distinct and functionally deviant; they embody direct and indirect threat (the risk of disease, the risk of social exclusion). The missing or distorted body part does not have to be visible, however, for the person who internalizes stigma, nor does she or he have to have experience stigmatizing behavior directly: she or he takes on cultural attitudes that give negative meanings to specific disabilities and incorporates these into unique ways of being in the world (Goffman 1963). Wearing a bag to collect urine or feces, and having to handle the bag and dispose of its products, provokes for many an internalized sense of revulsion that impinges on the most personal interactions, and presents a major barrier to establishing and sustaining personal relationships, as the preceding accounts of intimate relationships illustrate. Avoidance of others, for people with stigma, is one way to minimize disclosure and the risk of stigma. In many contexts, it proved unnecessary to discuss the stoma, and people maintained as much privacy as they could with outsiders as they went about their daily lives: hence the embarrassment with a public accident, when they were unveiled. But privacy is not possible in intimate relationships, for people with stomas must find a way of 'telling' a potential partner of the surgery, and to find ways to eroticize a body that is in some ways de-eroticized.

Sexuality and social life were especially problematic for single men and women, who were uneasy about meeting new partners and having to disclose that they had a stoma. Bubbaloo's experience after a colostomy was particularly extreme. She was in her early 30s when she had surgery for Crohn's disease. Her account captures a number of themes – inability to come to terms with surgery, followed by rationalization and a discourse of normality that made sense of her own responses as reflective of what "most people do." Bubbaloo was involved with someone at the time of her surgery:

> I was in a relationship, and when I knew that I would have a thing hanging off my stomach, I quickly just said, "Well, go, go and get a life," you know, just pushed him right out of my life. And I withdrew totally for five years. It was like going through a grieving period for about five years. I just felt dirty, I felt disfigured like you would not believe. I didn't want to know about it [the stoma], I didn't want to look at it, and the only reason that I even learnt how to maintain it was that I was told in hospital, if you don't know how to look after it you will never get home. I hated it. I just hated myself. There is no other way of describing my feelings. I was just beside myself, and I didn't like myself at all…. It is just the fact that you have got something hanging off your stomach that is full of weight. I went ten years without a relationship. I didn't feel worthy. At that point of my life, I just didn't feel worthy. My self-esteem was shattered. In those days, um, I'd been having a very rich life and good times. And all

of a sudden it wasn't there. I guess it was still there but I didn't feel part of it any more. I just didn't feel like, I was shattered, absolutely shattered. And I suppose the worst thing anyone can do is to withdraw like that and not let people in. I mean, I had people, a couple of friends in particular, who used to come and knock on my door, rattle the gate and goodness knows what, and I just couldn't even answer it, in case they were there and I had to go to the toilet or empty the bag. I'd listen for the car to pull away.

Bubbaloo spent five years after surgery virtually secluded, without any close friendships and rarely leaving her house, refusing to dine out, go to the movies, or meet new people. Ten years later, however, she met a man. He had no difficulty with the stoma:

> We had become sexually attracted to one another, I'd say, just in small ways, by walking together and brushing close, body touching, that sort of thing. And we made love….You read about all sorts of frilly underwear that you can buy that might sort of hide the fact (that you have a stoma), but if you want to be undressed then all the frilly pieces in the world aren't going to really do the job, I feel. I think I was carried away with the need to have sex and obviously he wasn't repulsed by it…. And we were able to have very satisfactory sex. I suppose I regretted that I didn't have 'the perfect body' any more. I may never have had 'the perfect body,' but certainly it's a very intimate sort of thing. He just didn't care about it at all. He used to say something about the bag, sometimes, and I would say, oh, don't say that. And I still am a bit like that. And I always wear a nightie, across here. I've sent away for everything that I have ever read was available.

Jane similarly had felt uneasy about establishing a sexual relationship, although her revulsion of the stoma was compounded by years of deprecation by her mother, embittered that her life course had diverted to caring for a sick child. Jane had to self-catheterize from early childhood. At the age of 13, she lost a kidney, and three years later, she had a colostomy. Her perspective of her surgery and the stoma, and her understanding of the relationship of the appliance to her reception as a person, highlight the social challenges for people when they must self-consciously manage their bodies:

> It's hard to live with, but I suppose it's better than being sick or incontinent. I had my kidney removed. That doesn't bother me as much as the colostomy, you know. You really basically feel disgusting. It surprises me still that my boyfriend accepts me for what I am, and doesn't

look at my body and think it's absolutely disgusting. On our first date, his big confession was, "By the way I am wearing contact lenses and I usually wear glasses." I never believed anyone could actually love me, I think. I feel it's legitimate to be depressed about it; I don't know. It's just hard sometimes.

Other men and women were relatively liberal, and refused to let the stoma interfere in their intimate lives. Vanessa, for instance, had an ileostomy after years of pain and diarrhea from ulcerative colitis, and she made up for any sexual constraints thereafter. One relationship, she recalled, was with "a Vietnam veteran who'd had both his legs blown off. We made an amusing sight in bed and understood each other very well. The bag leaking can be a pest though if it happens in someone else's bed. One night the bag flew off at the height of passion, and it went everywhere. But we were some sight – no legs and a bag."

Roger was impotent after a urostomy. But reflecting on sexuality and body-image, and describing in explicit detail his self-acclaimed talents in bed, he spoke of masculinity as "an ephemeral thing …something you don't have to prove, you've either got it or you haven't. In my case, I've got enough masculinity. I can still in a way give women pleasure, lots and lots of pleasure. I just can't give them intercourse. Now to some women that's a problem but, there again, that's their problem, not mine."

No part of the body is divested of all physical interests without severe psychical repercussions. Human subjects never simply have a body; rather, the body is always necessarily the object and subject of attitudes and judgments. It is psychically invested, never a matter of indifference. Human beings love their bodies (or, what amounts libidinally to the same thing, they hate them or parts of them). The body never has merely instrumental or utilitarian value for the subject. It is significant that the investment in and the various shapes of different parts of the body image are uneven. (Grosz 1994: 81)

The accounts of men and women with stomas of how they learn to deal in new ways with normal body functions, and to negotiate their bodies in general and particular social spaces, highlight the fact that bodies are ever present and dense with meaning. We engage with our bodies, unremarkably and imperceptibly, most of the time. We are always doing, using and interacting with our bodies, unintentionally and intentionally. Certain changes to the body sharpen all of the senses. A stoma is one such change: body functions and the signs of function are literally brought to the fore and imprinted with cultural meaning. Sounds, odor, texture, volume are all given an immediacy that is also a warning: body functions such as elimination can only be taken for granted because they are controlled. Out-of-control people must attend to their bodies constantly to prevent greater social disruption.

Notes

1. On their initiative, I interviewed a few people who had had stomas since childhood as a result of spina bifida or congenital defects of the urogenital system (e.g. bladder extrophy) or bowel (e.g. short bowel syndrome). Most had surgery after some years of managing incontinence, and other than the timeline, their accounts, experiences and perceptions were no different from those who had stoma surgery as adults.

2. The focus on specific health conditions in this volume has proven felicitous, ensuring the anonymity of individuals by presenting them in relation to a condition without fuller personal histories. This is a perpetual dilemma in anthropology and in other disciplines where substantial use is made of narrative or other qualitative data, where context is important both for representational and interpretive purposes.

3. In statements such as these, I am always reminded of Vieda Skultans's account (1970) of a Welsh informant, who explained that menopause made women more like men, thereby preventing them from undertaking such womanly duties as housework.

4. See also Merleau-Ponty 1962; Grosz 1994; Weiss 1999.

5

The Feminine in Question

Breasts are, as Iris Marion Young famously claimed, "the primary things" (1990:190), not only in the objectification of women but also, in multiple ways, as icons of womanhood. The breast is the flesh that nurtures, offers reassurance and comfort; an infant's embodied memory is buried long after the last suckle. Breasts are matters of beauty and pleasure, sex and sexuality, flamboyantly exposed in fashion, represented and admired in art, omnipresent on screen, discretely exposed with breastfeeding. Contemporary femininity, in its popular construction, gives breasts center stage. Recognizing this, the media invites public commentary on women's bodies in unparallel ways through the display of and judgment about screen idols who have had cosmetic surgery and who continue to aspire to be fashionable and desirable by displaying their flesh. In these contexts, the breast is highly visible. With disease, the breast is disconcertingly absent.

Worldwide, diseases of the breast are among the most common diseases that affect women. In Australia, around one in eleven women develops breast cancer. It is profoundly disruptive, its diagnosis auguring complicated personal responses, psychological reactions and extended treatment paths. This has generated considerable research and advocacy in comparison with other conditions. A large corpus of fiction, autobiographical writing and poetry, and visual artwork also exists, much of it by women who have turned to creative media to explore their own sense of bodily disruption and loss. Breast cancer is a rallying point for health activism and health promotion, both to raise funds for research and to encourage individual women to self-examine and present regularly for mammography to ensure early diagnosis and treatment (Figure 5.1). This suggests a level of popular awareness of the disease comparable only with HIV/AIDS. Yet despite its prevalence, there is still silence around both the disease and the body after cancer.

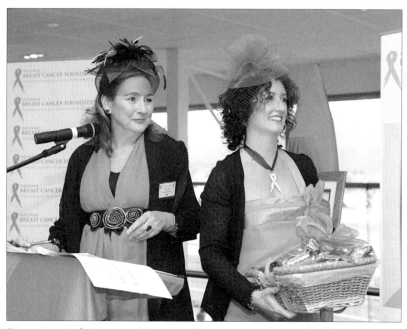

Figure 5.1 Judy Benson, Mistress of Ceremonies, and Judi Adams,
Chairperson, Think Pink Race Day, Hobart; 2010. Photograph by Tony
McKendrick. Courtesy of the National Breast Cancer Foundation.

In this chapter, I consider how women who have had a mastectomy
reconstruct themselves as gendered and sexual, in light of their history
of disease and the consequent absence of a breast or breasts. The loss of a
breast and adaptation to a body without a breast is particularly traumatic, because of the links between corporeality, gender identity and sexual
expression. Breast cancer exposes the vulnerability of any woman to her
body and the diseases that may attack it. The silence around breast cancer
is the silence of fear. I begin with Jill's account.

Jill found a lump in her left breast in 1992, while relaxing in a bath. She
came out of the bathroom and lit up a cigarette. Her partner admonished
her: "The way you smoke, you're going to die of lung cancer." She laughed
and said, "Well, I've just found a lump actually." Two weeks later, she was
in the hospital, comforting her concerned friends by insisting she had only
a cyst. A week later, however, she was asked to return to see the surgeon
to discuss how to manage what was now considered to be complicated
cancer. Jill agreed to a lumpectomy and then radiotherapy. Following the
lumpectomy, however, she was advised to have a full mastectomy because

the surgeon had been unable to excise all cancerous tissue. In reaction, Jill left the hospital, booked into a hotel, and as she tells it, rang up "everybody" in Australia to ask them their view about cancer and to discuss whether she should have her breast "cut off." Having done so, she returned to discuss this with the specialist. His advice was that she "might be able to keep the breast for a year or two, but that's all." Jill took the option and its implicit risk, and left.

Three months later, when she returned to the hospital for tests to get the 'all-clear,' she was advised to have a mastectomy immediately. Her task now was to arrange for reconstruction at the same time, as "there was no way I could wake up without a breast. I was 34 and single as far as I was concerned, and I couldn't cope with it. I just couldn't imagine not having a breast." But reconstructive surgery was only a beginning.

Eighteen months later, Jill woke up to discover that the prosthesis had deflated overnight: "I was looking in the mirror and this thing had shriveled up and it was like I'd had the mastectomy the day before. And it was only at that point that it clicked in my head, I don't have a breast." Jill spiraled into "personal crisis" in relation to what she considered to be a personal inadequacy – her inability to accept the absence of a breast and her desire for an internal prosthesis:

> I started beating myself up about it: "Well, I should be able to live with one breast, what's wrong with me? What does it really matter, am I really that superficial that I have to have two breasts?" So I lived without the breast, or with the breast all shriveled up, a bit of flappy skin hanging there with a shriveled up prosthesis for five months, trying to make this decision: will I have it done again or just have it taken out and live with the one breast? Eventually, I couldn't do it, I got a temporary prosthesis to stick in my bra, but I was always rearranging it; it wasn't satisfactory. So I opted for another reconstruction, but I felt weak somehow, I felt that there were other women who could handle living with one breast, and I wondered why I couldn't. I'd never seen myself as a superficial sort of person.... And I couldn't understand why I suddenly needed breasts when I'd never taken much notice of them before or even exposed them.

Jill decided to have a second reconstruction, which she said made her feel much better in mood, partly because the prosthesis was better: "I was more balanced, and it just seemed that it was easier to put on clothes and I did feel better." Yet still she felt confused, because her reconstructed breast was "not real": "I was tormented by the fact that I had no sensation, it was just sort of a numb part... I just, I was very angry and nobody wanted to hear about it much." Like many women involved in cancer activism, Jill began to 'paint out' her anger, taking advantage of the vehicle of expression with which she was most comfortable, putting onto canvas her experiences of diagnosis and surgery, and her ongoing fears: "I had this sort of thing of death hanging over me. *How much time, how much time?"*

Jill directed her energy to preparing a collection of works for an exhibition. But six weeks before the opening, five years after discovering the first lump, she found another lump at the edge of her nipple on the same (reconstructed) breast. Concurrently, she found a lump in her other breast. She was readmitted to the hospital. Her nipple on her reconstructed left breast was removed; she had a mastectomy with reconstruction of her right breast:

> I came out feeling I've got two numb nothings, but I can wear clothes and look normal. I felt like the top half of me was gone. *There was nothing, there was no sensation.* It was like half of my sex life had been taken away from me. If I drew myself, I would just cut myself off under the arms and resume from my navel. That's how I see it. I don't have any sensation behind my back here, either, it's completely dead. All my shoulder is dead, all around here.

For Jill, the absence of a nipple on one breast and the loss of sensation in both reconstructed breasts were constant reminders that the reconstruction was an illusion, inadequate to enable her to feel 'whole.' She found it difficult to "look at myself [i.e., her breasts]" in a mirror. Perception and appearance, the visual reinforcing the ideational, disrupted her sense of identity, with regard to both gender and rationality:

> I was surprised, because I didn't think that I needed both breasts. I always thought of myself as quite an attractive woman; I didn't stick my tits out or anything. I'm not a dumb blond but a woman in my own right. And now I'm embarrassed about it. And I'm angry at myself for being so pathetic. I haven't even, I thought that I'd accepted it; it's more like I'm resigned to it. You know, I've got scars everywhere. I don't even like looking at it because I look at it and I think mutilation, damage, defect, yuck.

Jill commenced radiotherapy and chemotherapy in 1998, and this added to her trauma. Nausea and vomiting following medical treatment underlined her sick despair at losing her breasts, as she battled first with a sense of disgust and horror at "being barbequed" and then, with agitated depression. She felt she was falling apart. She was frightened that if she started to cry, "it would be like pulling the thread of a jumper and I'd completely unravel." As her hair began to fall out due to chemotherapy, her agitation increased, complicated by an overwhelming sense of loss: "Handfuls [of hair] were coming out, but I wouldn't cut it. My hair was part of my sexuality and my femininity, and so it was the whole thing of, 'Okay the breasts have gone, now the hair. What am I now?'"

Painting Out the Pain

Creative work – visual art, photography, poetry writing, keeping a journal, making a quilt – provide people with a relatively unstructured way of working through emotions related to life-threatening illness and body loss, pain, grief and fear. In oncology programs, as in other programs for people who have experienced trauma, other life-threatening and degenerative conditions, and with psychiatric problems, art therapy can play an important role; it assists people to articulate their experiences and emotions in ways beyond the conventions of ordinary speech. As Scarry (1985) has argued, pain is beyond language; this applies very much to the psychological pain of people who face dramatic interventions to forestall life-threatening disease. The phenomenological approach in art therapy is that art promotes the act of 'seeing.' This, art therapists propose, is an essential ingredient that enables the person with cancer to gain objectivity, and concurrently, to address subconscious concerns about the disease and its trajectory (e.g. Deane, Carman, Fitch 2000:140). By doing so, art, as a therapeutic practice, helps people to find their own ways to deal with pain and misfortune. Even without tapping into the unconscious, creative work using any medium provides people with a way of 'talking' about their experiences.

Online art projects such as Breast Cancer Answers Art Gallery (1996–1999), Visual Aid, and Art.Rage.Us (1998, 2001) offer social support to transcend national boundaries. The works of artists contributing to these projects illustrate the raw pain and confusion that women experience with breast cancer.[1] Their art is seared with the intensity of emotion. Exhibitions bring people together. They are a means for women who have or have had breast cancer, and men and women who have cared for others with cancer, to tell a story that is both unique and shared, and by doing so, to enable others to bear witness, to memorialize, to find meaning in the experience, and to validate often overwhelming emotions of loss and grief. In these ways, they are transformative.

From January 27 to February 3, 2003, an exhibition entitled "Warrior Women" was held at Span Galleries, Melbourne; a second exhibition
of the work was held in the bayside city of Frankston in July that year.
Over the next year, "Warrior Women" traveled to eight more centers in
metropolitan and rural Victoria. The exhibition, sponsored by Breast Care
Victoria and the Victorian state government's Department of Human
Services, displayed the artwork of fifty individual women who had had
breast cancer, working alone or with other artists, and the joint work of
women from five breast cancer support groups. The exhibition included
written work – poetry, diary notes, non-fiction reflective pieces – and
visuals, including paintings, a slide show, montage, sculpture and videos.
Photographs and text dominated, however. These included collaborations
between professional photographers and community women with cancer;
most works involved some collaboration. One, a small graphic by Gisele
Pfab, was of a woman scaling a cliff, its caption reading, "She is still trying
to climb back to the top." Another work, on display when the exhibition
was at the Regional Art Gallery in Bendigo, Victoria, was by a local artist,
Denton Arthur: it depicted the single-breasted torso, photographed from
above and behind, a sensual fragmentary image of the artist's own body.
Other work at this exhibition made explicit the relationship between
therapy, support and personal resilience: one an open letter produced by
members of a support group; another a video of women using art therapy
to produce a quilt, as a way of coming to terms with cancer, stitching out
their anxiety and grief.

Other than Arthur's photograph of a torso, only one work depicted
bare breasts. This was *One in Eleven* (Figure 5.2) by Lurline Waters and
Sharon Jones, a large work which dominated the back wall of the Bendigo
gallery, dramatically making visual the epidemiology of breast cancer. A
photographic matrix of eleven by eleven breasts, one in each row (across
a diagonal from top left to bottom right) had been reshaped by cancer,
scarred, pocked, stitched, lopped and lopsided, or, in the last two rows,
reconstructed while the remaining breast was reduced.[2] Breasts without faces, anonymous objects disengaged from subjects, they could have
belonged to any woman, or the wife or mother or sister of any of the men
who entered the gallery. When I saw it, midday and midweek, people con-
tinuously moved through the space, forced by the detachment of breasts
from faces and hence from the biographies of particular people to gaze and
so acknowledge the possibility of cancer for any woman. That was its point.

Other photographs and texts captured women's experiences of the disease and its treatment: the confusion and pain of diagnosis and surgery, the shock of chemotherapy, the need to keep moving. Carmel writes of her loss of control over events, the "detour from life's superhighway … sitting in a dream … drowning … swirling in a whirlpool." Olga writes in the same vein: "When I first got breast cancer, it was as if my life was not directed by me anymore, but by some other force." As they write, women draw on metaphors of being naked, sexless, prepubescent, frightened, exposed. In one essay included as part of the project, also entitled *Warrior Women*, Annie writes of her shock after she had had a double prophylactic mastectomy because her mother had died from breast cancer at the age of 43 and her sister at 36, then to be diagnosed with breast cancer in the tissue remaining in her chest:

> The doctor says, "What you have is a little cancer." I focus only on several words "little cancer." What the fuck is a little cancer? Cancer is cancer. He mentions "good cancer" "early." These words do not console me. He is supposed to say "benign."

Meanwhile, Louise turns to humor to ground her experience:

> My first question was, of course, "Have I lost my breast?" The surgeon said, "Yes, we are very sorry." Then, as I have dentures, my next question was, "Can I please have my teeth?" When I look back, I have a little giggle to myself, because I was still suffering the effects of the anesthetic, and was lying so flat on my back [that] it took me several attempts to make them understand what I was trying to say, my mouth just seemed to wobble around like a block of jelly! Once I had my teeth back in, and a pillow, I was so very much more comfortable.

The production of art provides women with a voice and vocabulary to address their fear, loss and grief, and in doing so, to communicate this to others. The Victorian Anti-Cancer Council sponsored an exhibition by Melissa Jane Ades with this point in mind: her paintings are a visual diary of her experiences and dominant emotions, the anxieties, uncertainty, sadness and ironies of breast cancer.[3] The earliest painting from The Cancer Series, *The Wounded Woman* (1993), depicts a woman in a deep red slip, the left strap slipped from her shoulder to reveal the gaping hole that was once the site of her breast. She is gazing up at an angel-like figure, herself, waving, flying to the moon. In the background is a mosque: the painting, like others in the series, was painted while Ades was in Indonesia. In *Loss* (1995), a sad blue wounded woman dominates from the side, cradling her

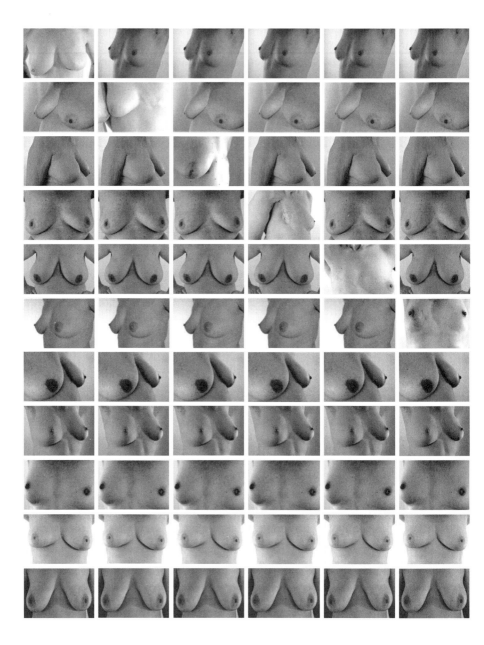

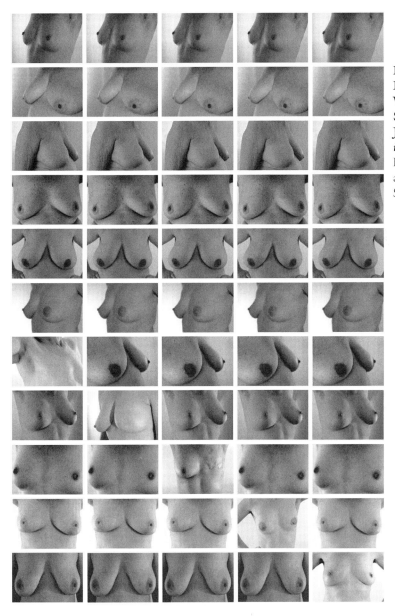

Figure 5.2
Lurline
Waters and
Sharon
Jones, *One
in Eleven.*
Photograph
and copyright:
Sharon Jones.

own scarred body. Beside her is another smaller figure, her face partly occluded, her hands over her mouth, a gesture of disbelief or horror. A figure, alive but corpse-like, hovers above; beneath it, small angelic figures illustrate divergent emotions: fear, anger, confusion, bemusement even. Murray (n.d.) suggests that the death that is depicted is of womanhood, of gender. In *Wholly Unable* (1995), the woman, now with an appalling gash from her hollowed chest to her vulva, is cradled by her partner; at the bottom of the painting, figures flee in panic. *The Second Sacrifice* (1996) (Figure 5.3), painted, on the suggestion of a friend, to revisit the pain and horror of the loss of a body part and sexuality, depicts the woman seated, cross-legged, alone. She looks both startled and confused. Her flesh is raw and ragged. Her mouth is an open O, echoing a scream from the O of the missing breast.

"Only a Breast, After All …"

The investments in and significance attributed to different parts of the body, and their contribution to an internalized body image, are not simply due to the subject's sensations or relations to others, but result also from the significance of body parts for others (Grosz 1994:82–83). Gender as a construct, and the relationship of flesh to gender, are somewhat abstract, but the flesh itself is anything but abstract. In chapter 3, I argued that the loss of a limb or the loss of a body function can be very public, and despite the best rehabilitation physicians and sophisticated technology, for the rest of their lives those who are affected will live and work with physical limitations. For this reason, I was surprised by the pragmatic responses and accommodation to impairment on practical, physical and psychological levels by those who had lost limbs, had had a stroke or had spinal cord injury: "I am normal … it's just that I have one leg" (Lynette); "You've just got to get yourself into normal habits with what you've got left and that's all there is to it. And not say, poor me, you don't think about it" (Jean); "I see myself as being normal again. I associate with these people. I am just one of the crowd. I am just myself" (Blue Boy). I assumed, too, that people who had lost bladder or bowel control, and who now had to manage elimination and waste consciously, would have difficulty with body image. As I illustrated in chapter 4, some people had great difficulty, leading them to reflect that they felt "flawed and inadequate" (Mia) and some – Daryl and Bubbaloo, notably – withdrew from social life for extended periods of time. Others, however, were pragmatic about the changes and

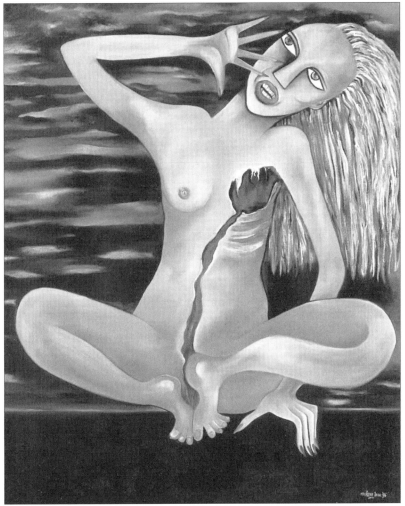

Figure 5.3 Melissa Jane Ades, *The second sacrifice;* 1996. Courtesy of the estate of Melissa Jane Ades.

the meanings these had for them; their sense of self was not tied to their bodily change: "I am normal ... it's just that I don't have a bum" (Dimity); "If anything, it's a novelty which can be ignored" (Vanessa).

In contrast, all women but one who had had a mastectomy described themselves as "not normal." Women spoke of having lost their "feminin-ity," the "wholesomeness of womanhood," or "woman's womanhood"; they said that they were now "not a complete lady" or "not quite the woman she was." Below, I draw on interviews in which women spoke of the impact of losing a breast in relation to their self-image and their being-in-the-world; and of the choices that they made with regard to using an external prosthesis or having reconstructive surgery. As will become clear, the weight of breasts, in terms of gendered identity, is substantial. The processes of diagnosis and treatment of cancer, and the meanings that women and their clinicians hold about prognosis, are beyond my concern here; I focus not on the disease, but only on the meaning of the presence or absence of breasts.

However, I want to discuss briefly women's responses to diagnosis, because of the ways in which they relate the diagnosis to flesh: the imagery of the disease as life threatening but also insidiously *in situ*. Women were shocked by the diagnosis, not because of the short-term implications of the management of the disease on their bodily integrity but because they were, with diagnosis, inevitability confronted with their own mortality. Roslyn, for example, reflected that the diagnosis was "devastating. When they tell you it's cancer, it's such a shock. You think that it's the end of the world, you know. Not that the breast had to come off, not that much. It's not that you grieve for the loss of the breast, it's more the shock of knowing you've got cancer." Anita likened the shock of diagnosis to being punched in the stomach: "It sort of takes your breath away, and you can't think." She continued: "The doctor is telling you that you're off work for the next eight weeks because you're having a mastectomy, and you have to say the words 'breast cancer' for the first time." Women were tearful as they recounted this experience, and as they described how learning that they had breast cancer spun them into a vortex of decision-making that was complicated by their fear of dying and its social implications, specifically their fear of not seeing their children or grandchildren grow to adulthood.

Yet in recalling their acknowledgement of the need to have surgery in order to continue to live, and their decision-making in relation to treatment paths, women recalled also their concern about the invasiveness of the surgery. Only a few women claimed that they did not worry about the loss of their breasts. Anita had had a lumpectomy, and five years later, after a recurrence of cancer, she had her breast removed. She felt that her breast was "*no longer necessary*. I could easily do without it and it would be one way of getting rid of a problem and preventing recurrence. I figured that was one part that I could easily do without; it didn't worry me in the slightest losing it. The cosmetic side of it doesn't worry me at all." Ann said that losing a breast hadn't worried her because she was so small-breasted that there wasn't much to lose; Maria and Roslyn both maintained that the thought of dying at the time of diagnosis and surgery overwhelmed all other emotions. Janice, too, reflected that she saw the "body as just a vehicle" and cancer a medical problem to be resolved; much later, her profound grief with regard to losing her breast surprised her:

> I got this image that the cancer's eating up an old coat or something, an old coat that I needed to discard anyway. It was eating me away. It was betrayal. It was, I felt, separate, too. I felt that my body was one thing and my spirit was another. I guess my first response to diagnosis was, "my breasts had cancer." It wasn't actually me.

Other women were mindful of the relative importance of their breasts to how they saw themselves and presented themselves to others, and this framed the decisions they made with regard to type of surgery and their responses to its outcomes. Erin opted for a lumpectomy the first time she needed surgery, for what at the time seemed to be practical reasons:

> Subconsciously I was thinking of the whole body image thing, I don't know. I said to the doctor, if you cannot convince me that having a mastectomy is going to give me a better chance of long term survival, then I don't need it. The quicker I can get out of hospital, the better. I mean, it's only a breast, after all. Only in the last year have I really realized that a woman's womanhood, whatever, femininity whatever, whatever word you want to use, really is defined in terms of her breasts and her uterus.

For Erin, it was not "only a breast, after all" – it was a breast dense with meaning. Meryl made a similar point with regard to both her breasts and uterus:

> I often wonder what part of our psyche is violated when you lose a breast, because you're very vulnerable without a breast. It feels like the wholesomeness of womanhood has been violated, and you feel less, you don't feel a complete lady, and of course you're not. Your breasts are important. And your womb: being married and bearing children, I know it's about the female role. They'll never get my womb; they'll never take that from me. Unwanted, but very much loved.

Stella took this imagery a step further. By losing a breast, she felt that she had lost a critical component of her femininity. She had bad dreams, she reflected, in which she was a man: "I'm a woman, but I'm just like a man."

As already established in previous chapters, men emphasize physical fitness and ability, while women more often equate self-worth with

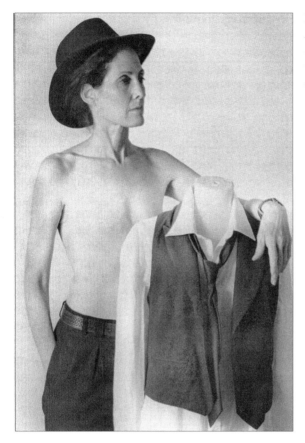

Figure 5.4
Ariela Shavid,
Self-Portrait; 1996.
Courtesy of Ariela
Shavid.

appearance and what they believe others think of their appearance.
Body ideals at any given time inform how women should or might wish
to appear, despite variations by class, culture and over time in relation
to weight and its distribution. It was striking, for instance, the number
of women who referred to their weight, particularly to being fat, and
regarded this as a greater concern to them, in shaping their body image,
than having a stoma or a prosthetic limb, for example. But breasts play
a particularly powerful role in body image, and the loss of a breast, the
resultant change in profile, and the scar tissue from mastectomy, all left
women disappointed, angry or depressed:

> I'd had major surgery previously; I did not want more mutilation. I
> made the decision to have the mastectomy very, very reluctantly and
> felt it was another great insult to the body that I was lopsided, and for

about six months, I'd say, I was angry and depressed. I think with the loss of a breast, there's some loss of femininity. I don't feel as though I'm as attractive as I was before the mastectomy. So that's a sort of perception. (Ruth)

The scarring from surgery, as depicted in *One in Eleven*, is significant both of itself and as a synecdoche. The visible disfigurement is ever-present, unable to be ignored and demanding either disguise or self-conscious accommodation. It stands for the disease and the surgery, but also, for the breast, femininity and sexuality. Women speak of "the scar" to refer to actual scar tissue, but also to the site of removal of breast tissue and as a synonym for "the absent breast" (Manderson and Stirling 2007). Women avoided looking in mirrors to avoid viewing the scar tissue and, in the absence of reconstruction, the concavity of their chest: "You look in the mirror and you see one side sunk in and the other side's not sunk in" (Evie). In the beginning, Ruth commented, "it's a shock every time you see yourself naked – you're maimed, you know." The visual reminders of surgery remain, and women liked neither to touch the scar tissue nor have it touched by others:

> It's a flat chest and there's a scar right across it. I suppose it's not all that gruesome but it took a while. It's a very silly thing but I kind of worried. It looked to me like a misshapen body, I suppose, and you keep telling yourself, after all you're alive, it's nothing really, but it does take a while to adjust to it. (Fran)

> Yeah, I've got a real problem with touching the scars. I mean as a woman with breast cancer, I'm meant to do self-examinations but I mean, very rarely. It's the breast cancer group that always says to me, have you done your … you know, touched yourself yet? And one woman in the group, when she looked, she just completely fell apart. She had a new husband, everything was all right in her life, really, but she just never actually had had a look, then she had a look and she was just horrified. (Julie)

Over time, women adapted to their appearance, but in discussing this with me, they were often embarrassed and apologetic lest they appear superficial by expressing their concerns with appearance: "I'm sure like most girls, I'm proud of my breasts. I didn't go around flaunting, I wasn't a superficial person. From my appearance I'm not the sort of person that goes around saying, if you've got it, flaunt it" (Lynette). How women come to terms with changes to their breast varies, however, and for some women, the sense of loss and disgust endures:

I see a shriveled-up nothingness, then I see the reconstruction, then I see the no nipple and the other one. I don't have a set image of myself anymore, I just see a series of chunks and bits and snippets and scars, and then because I'm quite visual in my mind, I see the whole thing flashing in front of me, it ends in nothingness. So when I look in the mirror, I don't actually look at my breasts because they're not there, or I'm in some serious denial, probably a bit of both. (Jill)

The image in the mirror is one, of course, that takes its meanings from society; it is not *merely* a reflection of a torso. In his observations on representation, Goffman (1959) observes that we perceive our bodies and our social selves as if looking in a mirror that offers a reflection framed in terms of (and shaped by) society's views and prejudices. Women build up an image of themselves in relation to their bodies, and deploy their bodies to project a particular image. In this context, women often referred to breast size when discussing adapting after surgery. Small-breasted women often assumed that it was easier for them than for full-breasted women to adjust, because they didn't "have enough to bother about because there was no shape" (Rocky); they speculated that if they'd been bigger breasted, the loss would have been more traumatic (Beverley). Eileen elaborated on this point:

> One of the reasons it didn't worry me is that I've always had very small breasts. It didn't feel like too much of a loss. I could understand the other women who were being hysterical with the real earth mother type big breasts – the earth mother goddess sort of person – but I never had that picture of myself. In fact, in a lot of ways I think I had a fairly masculine picture of myself. I was my father's boy until I hit puberty – that was the way it was. But it was also, I think until I had children, I was never sure that I was a complete woman, I suppose – I always doubted my femininity.

While Eileen did not anchor being a "complete woman" to having breasts, other women did so, and several recounted periods of profound depression following surgery and the loss of a breast as they began to question their femininity. A number of women had had radical surgery and had lost lymph nodes because of the invasiveness of cancer, and they had to come to terms also with additional problems of appearance and physical comfort associated with lymphedema. The removal of lymph nodes prevents the drainage of fluid and protein entering tissue from blood capillaries, and consequently the tissues tend to swell. Fluid retention prevents oxygenation of the tissues, thereby interfering with normal functioning, causing inflammation and inhibiting healing. Women with this condition had to wear compression bandages, massage and exercise, while they tried to reconcile themselves to bodily disfigurement and discomfort. Beverley held to the belief that in her case at least, lymphedema could have been avoided through more conservative surgery, and she felt that doctors underestimated its impact on women: "They just tell you not to worry about it, but it affects you for the rest of your life." Fran found it difficult because she lived in a tropical environment and the compression bandages were uncomfortable, and she found the time involved in exercise and massage demanding. In addition, the lymphedema drew attention to her, causing stares, glances of pity, and questions about breast cancer:

> I don't wear it [the bandage] all the time, but I should wear it. But people keep asking me why I'm wearing it, and I just say, "Oh, just to control lymphedema." And they go on, more often than not. They'll say, "What's lymphedema?" and kind of ask about it. And I know from the support group we're supposed to spread the word that everyone should be watching out for breast cancer and things like that, but I do find it difficult to tell people that I've had breast cancer.

Flesh To Hang On To

> *My existence is … a striving to hold together my schizoid being, to make the corporeality I am proud of and ashamed of in the fields of others coincide with the corporeality I am for myself – make that object there coincide with the here from which I perceive and extend my forces. (Lingis 1985:13)*

> *I still feel that breasts are part of the whole lovemaking act, aren't they? It's just that the imagery I get is that men hang on to breasts when you're having sex, right? And the image that I get is that when my partner … when we're having sex … he's got nothing to hang on to. (Janice)*

In writing in *Libido* of bodily subjectivity, Alfonso Lingis (1985) reflects on how an understanding of a body-for-others affects images of the self. The self is produced through interactions between the lived body (the body-for-me) and the body as experienced or perceived by others, and as re-interpreted or fed back to the individual; there is a continual feedback loop. Given the role of social interaction at the core of the social construction of the body, it is hardly surprising that people are so vulnerable and sensitive to bodily change, particularly when it has negative connotations and affects body parts such as breasts that are dense with social significance. Breast feeding and sexual expression both illustrate how breasts are a body-for-others. Corporeality is aligned with moral worth; dents in corporeal being eat away at a sense of self-worth.

Like men and women who have a stoma, women after mastectomy have to learn a new comportment, rearranging their bodies in space and navigating space in new ways, reflecting their heightened sensitivity to the possibility of pain through contact and their vulnerability to the recognition of difference were someone else (accidentally) to touch the mastectomized body. Women also spoke of literal disorientation; one woman claimed that she had lost a sense of balance with surgery, so that she now misjudged space and would bump into doorways. Others spoke of a heightened consciousness of the need to protect their bodies, particularly straight after surgery, to avoid "being knocked" or bumped: "You put up a shield with your arms" (Serena); "I put my arms in front of me covering my chest, because I just didn't want to feel pain any more" (Rebel). This self-consciousness persisted, and women reflected that in public especially, they choreographed position and movement to avoid being touched by others, to prevent injury but also disclosure. Women were self-conscious of the change of shape of their garments, too, worrying whether their top might be a bit too low, exposing scar tissue or indented flesh, or, if they had either an internal or external prosthesis, how their breasts flexed, flattened and folded or caved in ways that were different from 'normal' breasts.

In intimacy, the body post-mastectomy was especially problematic, requiring the most negotiation. Few women were able to discuss with their husbands, to their satisfaction, their feelings about having breast cancer and losing a breast, and few were comfortable being seen naked, their scarred chests exposed. Some women, like Wilhelmina, were reluctant to talk to anyone about cancer –"That's my way of coping and I coped quite well afterwards." Others were reluctant to discuss the disease out of concern for intimate others, because of their sense that an open discussion would heighten others' anxiety about prognosis and loss. But women were also reluctant to speak about breast cancer because of self-consciousness: "I know I was probably more worried for him than I was for myself, I think. The idea of cancer, I was talking about. But I really haven't sort of showed – I suppose I'm still very conscious of not having a breast there" (Marilyn).

Fran said that her husband had not shown any reaction to her breast loss, and had been "very sensible that way," but she also remarked that she always wore a nightdress and he rarely saw her undressed. Lynette used to dress and undress in the bathroom out of her husband's sight, "not let him in the bathroom, whereas (before surgery) we'd always moved in and out freely and not worried about things like that." Furthermore, a number of women were concerned that their husbands would reject them as sexual partners. As Beverley explained it, "your breast is part of being a woman I think, and you wonder what it's going to do to your married life." Roslyn reflected:

> I was aware that he was aware of it, you know what I mean? Because you've got no idea until it happens to you, if you've got big breasts and all of sudden there is nothing there, it's just your ribs, you know, it's a bit of skin over that big scar, so when you have sex, I was aware of it and I think my husband was, too, but he's always been very supportive.

Women's worries about being sexually desirable and sexual active were therefore partly a projection of what women thought their partners would think. Given the position of breasts in dominant ideas of women's sexual attractiveness, breast loss implied loss of desirability and desire:

> I think in the beginning months, I think maybe it did affect (our sex lives), not from his side but from mine. It was like, "Oh my god, I wonder what you must be thinking, I mean, how can you sort of still want me?" A turn off, you know what I mean, *that's how I was thinking surely he must be thinking.* But yeah, he didn't make a huge issue of it, he was really normal, he just was like, hey? I mean that was what it was about, it's not like the other part of your body which is just the same as it was before. (Erin)

Rena was the only woman who was able to move from self-consciousness to playfulness in relationship to her appearance and sexuality with her husband:

> I've got this concave (area) on my chest, and it's not a pretty sight. And that's how I felt. But Graeme just wiped those fears away because he's so kind. He's so understanding. It doesn't mean, those things, it's me the person that he really cares about and it just didn't matter. And you know, I'd rub up against him. The other night we were out and I was mucking around and I was edging up and I said, "It doesn't really feel like a no-boob, does it? It really feels like a real boob." And he said, "Can't tell the difference, can't tell the difference."

Rebel dealt with questions of sexuality and desire most directly. The intentionality of her surgery – elective bilateral prophylactic mastectomy because of her extensive family history of early breast, ovarian and other cancers – arguably provided her with the time and opportunity to discuss its implications with a genetic counselor, her surgeon and her boyfriend, time that women who had cancer usually lacked. Rebel was still revisiting her decision to have surgery as she was about to leave home for the hospital, and in recalling this in relation to conversations with her boyfriend, she reflected on her self-consciousness despite her intent:

> I said, "Are you going to be okay with this?" He said, "You need to do what you need to do to survive. It doesn't change who you are. If it's something you've got to do, then that's it, we'll work through it." Then the first time he stayed over after I came out of hospital, I just wouldn't switch on the light or anything. He kept saying, "Why don't you switch on the light?" I said, "I'm kind of embarrassed." He said, "What's to be embarrassed about?" I said, "Well, I don't feel normal." He said, "'Well, what's normal?" I said, "I don't know, it's just not the same." If we split, I don't know if I could do it again, you know, you've got to explain the whole thing and then you don't know whether that person is with you because they want to be with you or whether they're curious to see what it looks like, you know what I mean?

Further, like men and women who had had stomas, women who were comfortable with resuming sexual relationships often negotiated with their partners not to "intrude." Janice reflected that her husband didn't "press me about touching me in those areas where I've expressed like, I'd rather not," but she noted, too, that the result was a loss of erotic grammar: "there's nothing to hang on to." Eileen made it clear to her husband not to touch the scar: "I guess it reminds me that I am no longer a normal woman; I am mutilated. I guess if it's just all left alone then, I don't think about it." Finally, Serena, who had had a mastectomy for breast cancer and the prophylactic removal of the other breast, spoke of reinventing herself: "You make the most of what you've got and you just reinvent yourself in that way, the emotional side of it, the sexual side of it, you just get used to it. And you've got to be confident enough for everything."

Many of the women had reconstructive surgery. Almost all stressed that they had done so for their own sake, so that they felt normal. They emphasized that their husbands were often indifferent about them doing so or were concerned that their wives were choosing to have what they considered to be additional, unnecessary surgery. Women didn't see it like that: "Like now I can stand in the mirror. Although the breast is slightly different because it's smaller because of the infection, still it doesn't bother me. But before, it bothered me very much because you're maimed for life, you're not normal, you stand there and you're disfigured. It has to be nice" (Roslyn). Meryl was the only woman who said that her husband experienced difficulties with the mastectomy, and she had decided on reconstructive surgery for his sake rather than her own. Prior to the reconstruction, he would not look at the scar, he would not enter the bathroom if she were in it and undressed, nor would he make love to her unclothed. In recalling his responses to her after the mastectomy and then after reconstructive surgery, she illustrates how body image and sense of self are imparted and reinforced:

> I always had to wear a nightie in bed and my upper body had changed. I can remember my husband one night. It took him a while to work out which side of my body he could hold and which side he couldn't. I remember just feeling his hand hover above my left breast that wasn't there, and he pulled the hand away. So perhaps I didn't fully understand the adjustments he was having to make. But I understand that for some husbands, the scarring is there and it is a problem. It made me more convinced than ever to go ahead with the reconstruction, if not for me, for our relationship. I can walk naked in front of him now and he doesn't notice anything.

Taking Control

People with bodies that deviate from the norm – lack symmetry, are scarred, or in other ways are anomalous – are subject not only to stigma, as described in previous chapters, but also to the "relentless exertions (of others) to fix them" (Longmore 1997:153). "Disability," Longmore argues, "reassures Americans [and others] that they can still transcend the human condition. Thus, fixing disabled people has become a cultural imperative.… All they have to do is take people with disabilities and make them over" (156).

The imperative of 'making people over' is explicit in plastic surgery. Prostheses provide an illusion of the same process: the disabled appear able, the abnormal normal. Prostheses disguise – a false eye, for instance, covers an empty socket, a prosthetic breast disguises the excision of a diseased breast – or they minimize the impairment, sending a message of 'normalcy' to others despite evidence to the contrary. Reconstructive surgery takes this a step further. A reconstructed breast creates an illusion that there has been no change at all; the disease and the surgical amputation are erased.

While physiotherapy after breast surgery is intended to restore movement and flexibility to the arm and shoulder, and to manage lymphedema, and occupational therapy and counseling to address psychological aftereffects, rehabilitation also addresses practical questions. These include choices about prostheses and reconstruction. In choosing one or the other, women may respond in a way consistent with the socially overdetermined role of breasts in the constitution of female beauty, but also in a way that allows them to reclaim their own pre-illness status: to resist the label of 'cancer patient' and reaffirm their lives. As I illustrate, individual women sought to control their bodies by attempting to re-establish what they regarded as their former relationship with their body, while seeking to resolve the discordance between wanting control over their bodies and being unable to achieve this. I first consider how women use an external breast prosthesis to establish temporary symmetry, and then contrast this with women who decide to have a reconstruction and so create a more thorough illusion of body order. The choice of reconstructive surgery reveals much about individual women's attitudes about their breasts. Those who most insistently define themselves as female by their breasts were most likely to seek to keep their breasts through lumpectomy or reconstruction at time of surgery, for instance, or to re-create their breasts as a way of stabilizing a frail and fractured identity.

Rosenbaum and Roos (2000:153–154), drawing on the narratives of three women who had had breast cancer, highlight the pervasive ways in which women are evaluated by their appearance for much of their lives, how their appearance is defined significantly by their breasts, how treatment for breast cancer compromises their appearance, and therefore, how this troubles their identity and undermines their sense of self-worth. A compelling reason for a prosthesis, therefore, is not for the convenience of clothes hanging neatly, but because the symmetry of a two-breasted body ensures everyday social ease, public invisibility, and the avoidance of stigma. While a politics of breast cancer might resist the use of prostheses, their absence drawing attention to the underlying epidemiology of one in eleven (one in eight in the U.S.), women usually found it hard to talk about having had cancer, disliked the scrutiny by others of their bodies, disliked disclosing their experience, and were, as reflected above, self-conscious about scars, swelling and related blemishes. A number of women had dealt with stigmatizing behavior and were reluctant to place themselves in a continued position of vulnerability. Meryl, in particular, had difficulty because of her husband's revulsion by her breastlessness, but some women also were unsettled by other people's social unease. Many women reflected on the warmth of friends, but many also described how, seemingly suddenly, friends would cease to want to have lunch or spend time together. One woman spoke of friends who "just don't want to come anywhere near me," and others spoke of "the good friendships that I've maintained despite the surgery." Sharon had recurrent breast cancer from 1986 to 1997, including during pregnancy and breastfeeding, and she ended up with very different friends from those she had when she first found out she had cancer. She and other women described being "passed over" for nomination to attend workplace training courses because they "might not be around" subsequently, were not encouraged to attend conferences, and were not supported for promotion. Disguising surgery, or minimizing its seriousness by the illusion of a breast, was one way to reduce negative reactions from colleagues and other non-intimates. Women said as much, but also spoke of the impact a new breast could have for them:

> So to get over that, it [reconstruction] was a way of convincing myself that I was still alive and I was still going to live. It was me trying to grasp my life back again, get back into the land of the living if you like. And the only way to do that was to have my breast back. (Lynette)

Roslyn reflected on how important it was to her that the woman from a support group who visited her in the hospital was "just as big as me, probably even bigger." She showed Roslyn how to wear a prosthesis and made her a temporary prosthetic breast "from very soft material to put on when I went home under my nightie, because the big cut, it's sensitive." This had an immediate effect: "When you walk out of the hospital, you think that the whole world is staring at you because you've got nothing there, but if you put this [pad] there [in the bra], you know, that sort of support was so marvelous, was absolutely fantastic." Fran also chose to be fitted with an external prosthesis and commented on how much better she felt as a result. She supposed that it was because she "just looked normal again." Beverley chose an adhesive prosthetic which she felt was "a bit expensive" but "very natural looking." Like many women, she spoke of the extensive period of time that it had taken her to feel reconciled to the loss of her breast, and to feel sufficiently comfortable to walk around in her own home without

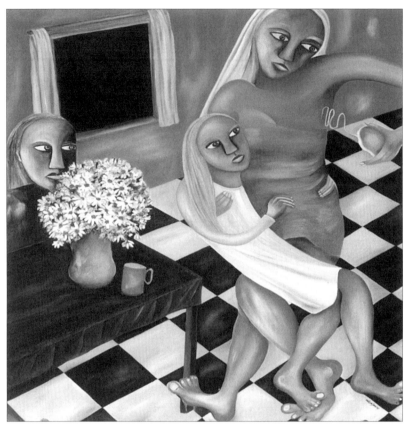

Figure 5.5 Melissa Jane Ades, *The external prosthesis;* 1997. Courtesy of the estate of Melissa Jane Ades.

covering up and without feeling embarrassed. The prosthesis helped her feel less self-conscious in more public spaces; by looking normal to others, she felt 'normal' to herself. But this is the public image. In *The External Prosthesis* (Figure 5.5), Melissa the cancer survivor holds her daughter as she juggles a prosthetic breast; Melissa the nurturer watches anxiously: Melissa the subject of the painting becomes a juggler, managing a cyborg body, sustaining a family, worrying about the future, fearing the worst.

The use of an external prosthesis was not common among women in this study, and most women took one of two other options. The first was an implanted prosthesis. For this to occur, a temporary saline expander is inserted under the chest muscle either at the time of the mastectomy or at a later date; when the breast tissue expands sufficiently, the pros-thesis, made from silicone and filled either with saline or silicone gel, is inserted. The other option was to have a breast reconstruction with tissue transplantation, using tissue from the abdomen, buttock or lat-eral thigh either pedicled or completely separated and reattached to the chest with microsurgery, with darker skin from the inner thigh used to construct a nipple. The decision to proceed with reconstructions was rarely simple. Ruth, for instance, was conscious of debates about agency and social pressure, and the extent to which by having a reconstruction she was complicit with sexist social values: "I've heard other women say, I don't care – one tit, two tits, what does it matter? But I would think most women would feel it's an assault on their body to have that bit cut off and thrown in the bin. I sometimes think: 'What did they do with it, did they just burn it?'"

Ruth's decision to have a reconstruction occurred after she had worn an external prosthesis for some time. She had been happy with the prosthe-sis initially, but found it uncomfortable in hot weather and she developed a rash. In explaining the decision to have reconstructive surgery, however, she spoke of both self-image – "one great big cut-off" – and lack of moral strength; she described herself as very "self-pitying":

> If I'm gardening, bending over, it [the external prosthesis] sometimes falls out, and that's very off-putting. I've met women who've had a mastectomy perhaps twenty-five years ago – small-built women per-haps who have just stuffed a couple of tissues down their bra and not been aware that you could even get a prosthesis; nobody's ever told them. And other bigger built women who've stuffed a sock or a couple of socks into their bra. I just felt very dissatisfied with my whole lot in life and presenting my body with one great big cut-off and somebody measuring me to try and find a bit that might fill in for the bit that was cut off. And I suppose I felt I was being singled out as, "this must be a woman who's lost a breast because she's going into that particular shop, and coming out with a big box under her arm." It was a general shop selling lingerie but it also specialized in prostheses. I was just very, very sorry for myself and very self-pitying and possibly physi-cally run-down – just physically and emotionally unwell.

Roslyn also delayed having a reconstruction. She chose to do so two years after the mastectomy, despite fear of the procedure and pain, because it would be her own body, "just transferred from here to there, you know, so everything is yours. I know my body doesn't feel different – it's mine, you know, it's back to normal so to speak." She took this choice after she met with and was able to look at the breasts of another woman who had had a reconstruction on one side and a reduction on the other: "it was beautiful, it was perfect. She was like normal again, you know, because that's the feeling, you're not normal if you've got one big breast and nothing on the other side. Well I did, I felt very [self-]conscious."

Thus, even women who were relatively pragmatic were also influenced by a sense of not being normal, as understood simply in terms of their difference from the majority. Other women linked their decision-making to social participation. Erin, for example, wanted to be able to undertake a range of usual activities. She had had a lumpectomy rather than a full mastectomy, but as she described it, "the nipple's still there but not much else." She was particularly self-conscious when she went swimming, because she felt that people stared at her, curious about her mastectomy and conscious of being curious: "It's a common sort of curiosity, you wonder what it looks like, you know." And, as noted above, Meryl had a reconstruction because of her husband's rejection of her body after surgery:

> You feel so whole. I felt whole again. It was wonderful. I even had a nipple. And I believe they do them much better these days, mine's gone flat. I don't tell many people this, but I'm like a patchwork quilt because they take bits from here and bits from there and I have scars under my arm, my groin, across my back.

Lynette's choice to have reconstructive and reductive surgery provides another example of the complex ways in which women experience their bodies. Home from breast surgery for cancer, Lynette used to get out of the shower in the morning and weep, "confronted by this strange woman, not only with a breast missing, but with a concave breast on one side because the muscle had been eroded so badly by the surgery. And a fairly large breast on the other side." In her words:

> I put up with this for quite some time and then eventually I thought, I've got to do something about this and I wanted to have something done to remedy the situation, because I wanted my breast back, I couldn't accept, I couldn't stop grieving the fact that I'd lost my breast. And I don't know why, because I'd never been that sort of a person. It's a long story because so many things went wrong. I was in search for my breast, because really that's what it was, I was searching and I wasn't prepared to give up until I had it back.

At the same time that she had an internal prosthesis, Lynette had a breast reduction. This breast became infected, and nearly required amputation. She had numerous problems with the prosthesis, too, and finally, almost three years after the original surgery, she had it removed and replaced. Now, she comments, her husband will sometimes put his arm around her and have his hand on her new breast and forget, unless she reminds him that he's got his hand on the "wrong one." She worries that it might not feel the same, but she also says she would never have been comfortable with him putting his hand on her concave chest "because it really was an ugly mastectomy. Not the scar itself, just the appearance of it because it was just as I said, not a skerrick of tissue left." Yet despite surgery, Lynette still reflected that she had never recovered her confidence in herself "as a woman." As she concluded, "I don't know why, because there's no reason why you're any less of a woman for not having a breast. But if that's the way you have all of that in your head, there's very little you can do about it."

Two women in the study, introduced earlier, had breast reconstructions after a prophylactic mastectomy. Serena had breast cancer and a lumpectomy in one breast at the age of 34. After it was established that she was at risk genetically, she had a full bilateral mastectomy and silicone reconstructions. Rebel had not had breast cancer herself, but at 29, again in light of family history and positive results from screening, she decided to have both breasts removed and reconstructive surgery with implants. Both women were adamant that they would not have had surgery unless they were absolutely convinced of their probability of developing breast disease, both found surgery and especially reconstruction painful, and neither would have considered mastectomy without reconstruction. Serena had decided not to have a reconstruction when she first had surgery for breast cancer. But subsequently, she decided to have internal prostheses both because of how she felt about *herself* – "I just want to be me again" – and about feeling feminine, even though, contradictorily, she also felt she was no longer "the woman that she was" because she no longer had her *own* breasts.

> What's femininity? You could start anywhere. Every woman will define it in her own way. But it's a confidence thing. It's a control thing. I am a woman and with these [breasts], I can get you. It's that sort of thing. It's a take-charge thing. I look good, I feel good, but without these, I don't feel 100 percent. It's not me, it really isn't. It's not the breasts or your face or all these things, it's the person that you are. I

have dug deep and soul-searched and all those things and, yes, day by day you'd get by, but I'll always stand by the fact that without breasts, you're not complete. You've had the operation, and that's part of the fact of living or dying, but your femininity is gone, the woman that you are. It's part of being a woman for me. (Serena)

Rebel felt that she had no choice but to have prophylactic surgery, and she recognized that she was still at risk of getting cancer. She spoke of the impossibility of reconciling to the loss of her breasts:

If it's going to come, it [cancer] will come. So I can only try and prevent it from coming. I can't decide, "No, that's it, I'm not going to get it" because I carry the gene. So it could hit me eventually. I can only make a choice and have control over trying to stop it from occurring, but then again, who's to say that it won't? There's still that chance, whether you take precautions or not. And there's no point in waiting. You're never ready for that procedure. Not for a woman. That's your femininity, it's, I don't know, it's just part of who you are. And the last night I had my breasts, I concentrated hard on this feeling and sensation, so I could take it with me and remember it when I woke up.

Amazon Women

Coming to terms with bodily change after mastectomy includes making decisions about the post-surgical body. Kathy Davis (1995:157) maintains that in making a decision to have cosmetic breast surgery, women exercise agency, acting upon circumstances in a particular way to enhance their wellbeing. With breast cancer, this is even more the case. Attitudes about breasts and feminine identity provide a filter though which women relate to breast loss and the impact of this on their lives and identity (Rosenbaum and Roos 2000:166). As suggested, prosthetic surgery is one way to erase the embodied anomaly of breast loss. The erasure is a superficial one, of course; women do not forget.

In analyzing their emotional responses to the loss of their breasts and to making decisions about the use of prostheses or reconstructive surgery, women were often surprised by the intensity of their own feelings and by what they felt to be their own intellectual superficiality. While most women defined themselves as women, feminine and sexual in terms of their breasts, many were embarrassed or surprised that they found it impossible to dispense with social attitudes that objectified women and their bodies. A number of women had played with the idea of remaining

single-breasted, often using rather bleak humor in their attempts to come
to terms with loss:

> We had fun one day trying to think of all the advantages of only hav-
> ing one breast, like, if someone attempted to rape you they'd probably
> drop you in fright; if you're traveling overseas you have the ideal spot
> to hide your money; or you could buy a bra and cut it in half so it would
> last twice as long – we had quite a bit of fun trying to think of all these
> silly things. You have to look at the funny side of things. (Fran)

Other women were wary of the resistance involved in being single-
breasted from their own and others' viewpoints. Erin, for instance, felt
confronted by the very idea of being single-breasted, publicly exposing
her mastectomized body and so drawing attention to her experience of
cancer. In her work on performance art, Rosemarie Garland-Thomson
(1997a, 2009) draws attention to the politics of confrontation: by exposing her body and its congenital deformities, she challenges her audience
and prods at its biases. The political comportment of the body is common
in performance art, as I noted in relation to Annie Sprinkle's performance
(chapter 4). Raimund Hoghe's seductive dance performances, the denoué-
ment his exposure of his twisted spine, is a less familiar example (chapter
2). But Erin was neither a performance artist nor an activist, nor did she
wish to be, and her perceived need to protect others from the ravages of
cancer, and to spare herself and them from their revulsion, says much
about how cancer, but also other diseases and death, remain stigmatized
and continue to unsettle.

> I think that I would feel self-conscious and I think that other people
> would feel uncomfortable. It really does look ugly. It looks completely
> abnormal. And I think a lot of people know you've had cancer, but a lot
> of them don't know and it's one of those issues, do you talk about it or
> don't you, do you know what I mean? I just don't want other people to
> feel uncomfortable about it, you know. I have a little bit of admiration
> for women who are able to identify as breast cancer survivors, who
> talk about throwing their prostheses away and just going, what the
> hell and going on a camping trip and stripping and, you know. And
> I think that must be extremely liberating for them and I think that's
> fabulous, but I have a huge problem about whether other people feel
> comfortable with that. I have a real problem with other people hav-
> ing to be confronted with stuff that they probably really don't feel like
> dealing with. (Erin)

Anita was not self-consciousness about her prosthesis, but again, she was aware of the way in which the visible evidence of cancer might disturb others: "I've got over it. Sometimes I forget to put it [my prosthesis] on and I race back upstairs, like I did this morning. It doesn't worry me not wearing it, but I think it just saves other people's embarrassment by having it on. My sister doesn't even notice it if I've got it on or not." With encouragement from others in her breast cancer support group, Anita now introduces herself as an Amazon woman.

In examining medical, social and fictional narratives of the English Renaissance, Kathryn Schwarz (1997:147–149) describes the use of the female breast to reify women as erotic objects and as objects of domesticity and vulnerability to disease. In describing this, she refers to the mythologized Amazonian body, imagined through the absence of the breast, in which women have actively rejected their feminized sexual and maternal roles. The Amazon woman is androgynous; she has traded the social and personal rewards/obligations of maternity, wifehood and motherhood with personal freedom. Poet Audré Lorde recalls this mythology when she identifies herself, post-mastectomy, with the Amazons.[4] So do Anita and her friends. Women who resist reconstruction, and tattoo their chests post-operatively, acknowledge the signification of the breast. But the tattoo is an unnecessary reminder for those who have had cancer; the scar tissue and flat chest is mnemonic enough. And as Lorde notes, "When I mourn my right breast, it is not the appearance of it I mourn, but the feeling and the fact" (1980:65). Again, it is artists – poets, painters, photographers, including women who only became artists because they had had breast cancer – who have access to the technology to question the centrality of breasts to women's identity by their self-reflection. In this concluding section, I return to art to explore the work of artist-survivors who pursue the idea of the Amazon body through representations of their own body and experiences.

The iconic photograph of Deena Metzger by Hella Hammid, c 1978, of her mastectomy scar tattooed as a branch with leaves, is the starting point of warrior women and resistance photography. Subsequently, from the cover of *The New York Times Magazine* in 1993 (Beauty out of Damage), Matuschka's photographs illustrated the point at which "the exposed mastectomy scar went mainstream" (Anonymous 1998; Ferguson and Kasper 2000; Lerner 2001). The photograph of supermodel Gisele Bundchen wearing the logo of the Fashion Targets Breast Cancer campaign in 2003 built on this symbolism, and again the imagery challenges conceptions of female beauty as necessarily two-breasted and unblemished. While artists such as photographer Jo Spence challenge cultural notions of femininity in self-portraits that show a body "middle-aged, irregular, [defying] the canons of ideal feminine" beauty (Davis 1997:63), Matuschka and lesser known Israeli artist Ariela Shavid have challenged these notions from the starting point of conventional, fashionable beauty; in their work the viewer/voyeur is faced with single-breasted beauty (see Figure 5.4 above).[5]

Shavid's exhibition and installation *Beauty is a promise of happiness* opened at the Israel Museum in Jerusalem in 1996, in Paris in 1997, and again at the Tel Aviv Museum in 1998, to critical success and to moving personal responses from those who saw her work (Dovev 1996).[6] The frontispiece of the catalogue (the Hebrew, not the English, front) is Zurbarán's *Saint Agatha* (Zurbarán 1630–33) proffering her amputated anachronistically rather silicone-like breasts on a platter, surrendering sexuality and gender to give herself, with virginal devotion, to Christ.

Shavid's own work is mixed media, with photographic self-portraits, prints, textiles and sculpture, with the playful use of the material culture of women's lives and contemporary commercial society. Her reflections regarding the exhibition explain how her experience with breast cancer and surgery "served as a springboard for dealing with questions of femininity, masculinity, loss, self-image and universal existence" (Dovev 1996:1). Shavid was born in Haifa, Israel, in 1945. After she completed her army service, she worked as a model, "an occupation that contradicted [her] feminist inclinations" yet gave her access to an incongruously glamorous world that had been symbolically represented in childhood by boxes of pretty hand-me-down dresses. She left modeling after a short period to study photography and cinematography, worked as a professional photographer until she married and had two children, established herself as a portrait photographer, and then studied social work. Her cancer illness occurred at the point at which she had decided to concentrate on art.

The exhibition of photographs and plastic arts explores the relationship of body to identity and follows from Shavid's own decision to eschew breast reconstruction. She recalls, "I woke up to reality and decided to examine … how I had come to internalize the 'Barbie' image that is so dominant in our society" (Dovev 1996:3). Shavid continues to ask: "What is the meaning of a sculpted breast that does not give sexual pleasure, that does not fulfill its erotic promise?… Why can't women walk around comfortably in clothes that show them as they are without the need to feel

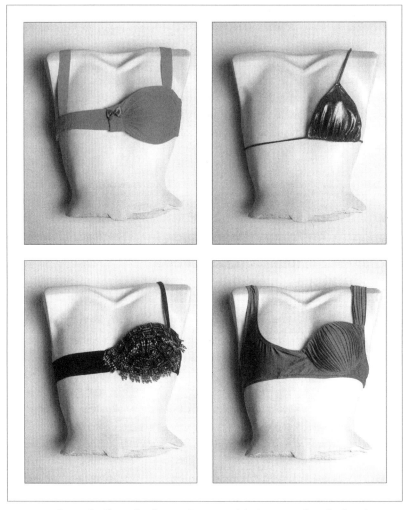

Figure 5.6 Ariela Shavid, *Plaster Casts;* 1966. Courtesy of Ariela Shavid.

shame and invent camouflages?" (3–4). She concludes: "This exhibition is not just about breast cancer. It deals with losses of all kinds, visible and invisible, physical and emotional – and with growth. It addresses questions such as the importance of the missing part of our life versus what is left" (4). Hence the powerfully seductive wet T-shirt calendar, one-breasted Barbie dolls, paper wardrobes for paper-doll Amazon women, the plaster casts of the female torso, its single breast adorned in luxurious bras (Figure 5.6), and embroidered felt self-portraits. T-shirts with printed scars were available for sale at the exhibition. There is a play with gender, too, in the black and white androgynous photographs of Shavid in suit and tie and in a second portrait, stripped to the waist, a Marlboro pack tucked into her waistband. This invites two, not exclusive, interpretations: the cigarettes as a symbol of masculinity (in keeping with the mirage of Shavid as a man) and of power, or a graphic epidemiological footnote, given the link between cigarette smoking and breast cancer. The theme is revisited in some of Matuschka's later photographs (e.g. *Which side do you want?* c.2001 and *I'm a woman,* c.2001).

Visual arts and other uses of media draw attention to the prevalence of breast cancer and the need for greater investment in research and screening. In the same way that the Warrior Women exhibition in Australia exposed breast cancer and its profound personal impact in one geographic setting, Shavid's work draws attention to the social and individual dimensions of the disease in ways that enhance local advocacy. The Israeli Breast Cancer Coalition was established by a number of community-based and feminist organizations in 1994 to address what its members considered to be a 'conspiracy of silence' surrounding breast disease, the particular reluctance of women from conservative religious communities to participate in screening programs, and the low profile of breast cancer on the national health agenda.[7] In 2006, the coalition continued to draw on Shavid's work to highlight the increased incidence of breast cancer in Israel, and to advocate for a greater commitment to screening, early diagnosis and improved care. While street marches and other public activities allow high profile advocacy, as the Coalition has pointed out, art has proven to be a particularly effective method of maintaining advocacy. In this context, the exhibitions of work by Ariela Shavid and others (Shuli Nachshon, Claudie Cobut and Boaz Tal) have all had marked impact on how women see themselves, and on the choices they believe they can make.

Notes

1. Visual Aid is based in San Francisco and provides assistance to artists with life-threatening disease, including by assisting artists with supplies, mounting public and on-line exhibitions and holding workshops, providing studio assistants, and maintaining an archive of visual and bibliography material. Numerous novels, biographical anthologies and catalogues of art relate to breast cancer (de Moulin 1983; Gawler 1994; Lossy 1996; King 1997; Anonymous 1998; Raz 1999; Bowes, Gingras, Kaplowitt, Perkins 2000; Kasper and Ferguson 2000).

2. Lurline Waters is a breast cancer survivor, Sharon Jones a photographer; both were members of the steering committee of "Warrior Women." The work contrasts with most of the other work included in "Warrior Women," which included portraits of women who would not have been otherwise identified as breast cancer survivors. It contrasts, too, with the autobiographic content and specificity of Diana C.Young's photograph *One in Eight* (1996): here the artist is shown with a mastectomy, in the company of six of her two-breasted friends, and the daughter of one of them (Eikenberry 1998). I thank Keely Macarow for drawing my attention to "Warrior Women," and Sue Smith for finding the images and digitally reconstructing the work for this book.

3. The exhibition *The Cancer Series* (Ades 1997) included paintings from 1993 to 1996. A second exhibition of the series, with additional work, was held at the Cato Gallery, Melbourne, in 1998; the work is to be shown in a retrospective planned for 2012. The paintings here are reproduced with permission of the artist's husband.

4. Lorde's comfortableness with this identification is supported by her prior public identity as a lesbian (as well as, in her own words, fat, blind and Black) and her embrace of the mythical associations of Amazon women with strength, masculine pursuits, and resistance to reproductive roles (Miner 1997).

5. Matuschka was best known as a model when the *New York Times Magazine* cover photo, of the mastectomy self-portrait (headlined *You cant look away anymore*, August 15, 1993) appeared. However, she had already, from 1972, worked with painting, drawing and photography, had a number of exhibitions in the United States and Europe, and begun prose, poetry and song writing. Her very funny and honest curriculum vitae ("Works as a cocktail waitress and starts taking drugs," "Quits college. Fired from taxi cab company.") is on her website at the time of this writing (Matuschka 2003).

6. I am indebted to Amalia Rosenblum, Ariela Shavid's daughter, who introduced me to her mother's work and gave me copies of the catalogue and Shavid's reflections on the exhibition, and to Shavid for writing to me in response to an early paper on which part of this chapter is based.

7. Israeli Breast Cancer Coalition, 2006. Address to National Breast Cancer Coalition Fund, 2006. Annual Advocacy Training Conference, Washington, D.C., April 29–May 2. http://www.natlbcc.org/bin/index2.asp?strid=259&btnid=5&depid=5; accessed May 31, 2006.

6

Replaceable Parts: The End of Natural Life

Your natural life has ended. You rely on machines to keep you alive.
(Rick, research participant)

An amputation is the most concrete example of the surface tensions that occur as a consequence of bodily change, as suggested in chapter 3. The absence of a limb is manifest to the person who has experienced loss, but, depending on dress style and site, more or less so to others in his or her social environment, intimates and strangers alike. But in their continuing relationships, intimates bring a studied appreciation of the meaning of amputation for themselves and the other; they have deliberated on the preconceptions, myths, fears and esthetics of embodied change and addressed in theory and in practice how loss can restructure intimacy. Strangers do not have the luxury of premeditation. When an amputation is visible through a noticeable prosthesis, for instance, the reaction of a stranger is shaped by pre-existing knowledge and prejudices about causes, and by readings of the body for supplementary clues. Age and gender, other bodily signs of health status, scar tissue, and race can all hint at the cause of the loss of a limb, albeit often in error, and so lead to presumptions about personal qualities and social worth. An amputated lower leg, for example, references different body histories according to age, style and appearance, even body weight, and provides an index of social location. Almost any disability provokes stares and shame (Garland-Thomson 2009).

Transplants involve but contrast with other amputations, because superficially, the corporeal changes of transplantation are indiscernible. This disguises the nature of body loss, reconstitution and surface tension; the lack of awareness of the 'amputation' or excision is true only from the standpoint of strangers. For the person who has had transplantation, his or her intimates, and the donor or donor family, the embodied changes are ubiquitous reminders of the various bodies involved, and of the ironies of transplantation and the vital persistent everyday actions of maintenance.

Like other cases in this book, transplantation is a constitutive moment in the body's history. The difference is its sequel – the use of another person's living tissue or organ to sustain the functions once undertaken by the organ now removed, or the organ left in but residual, no longer functional. Transplantation provokes introspection and reflection for various players through the multiple meanings ascribed to the surgery, the unique history of the body part or tissue, the relationship of part to whole, the subsequent surveillance of the body's workings, and the particular tensions of personhood.

The Development of Transplantation

Transplantation surgery has become increasingly controversial, particularly because of the mismatch between demand and supply, as anthropologists including Nancy Scheper-Hughes (2002a, 2000b, 2004), Margaret Lock (2001), Lawrence Cohen (2001) and Lesley Sharp (2006), among others, have described. But the technology and the demand for such surgery are not new, as again I show by providing a summary history of scientific experimentation and surgical developments. In doing so, I want to emphasize the preparation of the social ground by a scientific imagination for contemporary developments that include, diversely, immunological advances, surgical experimentation, and human rights abuses associated with organ theft.

Fantasies of organ transplants to extend life, like imagined external grafts to restore function and appearance that anticipated recent developments in reconstructive surgery, reattachment and transplantation, are centuries old. Moore (1964) maintains that the possibility of organ transplant dates at least from the thirteenth century, and surgeons reported nose reattachments from the sixteenth century (Williams 1971:415). The experimental work that took place in France in the eighteenth and nineteenth centuries illustrates an extraordinary interest in the power and possibilities of surgery and the relationships between mechanics and human life – analogical, transferable, replaceable, fantastic – such that the developments of the late twentieth and early twenty-first century appear, in context, to be entirely predictable (Wood 2002).

The first successful autograft, involving resiting and grafting skin on a sheep, was conducted by Baronio in Italy in 1804 (MacLean, MacKinnon, Dossetor 1971:67). A century later in France, Carrel was conducting research and publishing on experiments involving blood vessels, organs and limbs, undertaking the groundwork for human organ transplants. One of the earliest experiments was a heterotopic allograft, in which the heart from a donor dog was placed beneath the skin in the neck of another dog, with blood to the allograft supplied from the carotid artery (304). The allograft lasted a few days only, but long enough to fuel scientific optimism about the viability of same-species organ donation. In 1907, Carrel used this same procedure to transplant the lung of a kitten to the neck vessels of an adult cat; the following year he successfully transplanted a spleen in a dog, the beginning of years of work in search of a surgical answer to diabetes. Carrel and Guthrie also experimented with limb reattachment, and in 1908 reported a replanted dog limb that lasted for twenty-two days. Other laboratories were also experimenting with grafts, replantation and transplantation (Manax and Lillihei 1971), and research with dogs, then primates and humans, proceeded in fits and starts from this time on, propelled and interrupted by the two world wars. Successful skin grafts of identical human twins were first documented in 1927. The first transplantation of whole lung and pulmonary lobes occurred in a dog in 1947, and by 1950 a number of teams in France, the United States and the United Kingdom had successfully conducted lung transplants.

Human kidney transplant is the longest established and most prevalent organ transplant surgery. Experiments with animals were published from 1902 (Dahm and Weber 2002), and continued through the 1920s. By the mid 1930s in Europe and the early 1940s in the U.S., teams were reporting successful temporary human kidney transplants. The first successful orthotopic (i.e., in the normal position) kidney transplant, involving monozygotic twins as donor and recipient, was conducted in the U.S. in late 1954, and within a decade kidney transplants were being conducted relatively widely in major centers in Europe, Canada, the U.S., and from 1965, in Australia. By this time, too, successful human liver transplantation had elevated optimism about other possible transplant surgery.

Research in the early 1960s had established the compatibility of human and pig blood, and extensive experimentation had occurred to test the use of cadaver human and pig livers for temporary extracorporeal support. In 1966 and 1967, too, baboons with human blood were used as parabiotic partners of comatose patients with liver failure (Eiseman and Velasquez 1971:106–108), although by the 2000s the possibility of xenotransplantation using primates had receded because of the high risk of cross-species infection. Interest in xenotransplantation remained, however, because of the limited supply of cadaver organs and the insufficient numbers of compatible live donors, with the pig remaining a favored candidate organ donor because pigs are "physically quite similar to humans" (Pirani 2002), in terms of the comparable size of human and pig organs and the ease of breeding pigs if not in terms of its problematic cultural status. Consequent research has included the use of bovine and porcine tissue for vein grafts, hybrid liver support systems and islet (endocrine cell) transplantation for diabetes, among others, with concern specifically related to safety and the risk of cross-species infection rather than squeamishness about hybridity (Deschamps, Roux, Sai, Gouin 2005; Yang and Sykes 2007).

Other transplantations took place during this same period, again at a rather breathless pace from first animal experiments to routine procedure. Preliminary work for heart transplantation, for instance, was conducted from the mid 1950s, once a pump oxygenator had been developed to maintain oxygen supply to the blood while the vessels were being resutured. The first heart transplant was performed in South Africa in 1967, and within a year, 107 heart transplants had been undertaken in twenty-four countries by sixty-four teams (Lamb 1990). The first artificial heart transplant (Jarvik 7) occurred in 1982, and two years later, two-day old infant, Baby Fae, received a baboon heart. Pigs and baboons for liver transplantation had been taking place for some twenty years. The first heart-lung transplant occurred in 1981, and this was followed by multiple organ transplants: heart-liver, liver-kidney, pancreas/kidney/duodenum, and double lungs. Body parts frozen after severing can often be reattached with restored function, and consequently microsurgical developments have also been substantial. The first successful replant occurred in 1962, when the arm of a twelve-year-old, traumatically amputated below the shoulder, was reattached (Malt and McKhann 1964). The first recorded graft took place in Ecuador in 1964; without sophisticated immunosuppressive drugs, it was rejected two weeks later. The first successful hand graft took place in Lyon, France in September 1998, followed by a graft in Louisville, Kentucky, in early 1999, then in China, Malaysia, Italy and Australia. The first double-hand transplant was performed again in Lyon in January 2000, with subsequent cases in Austria and China. Complex tissue and limb transplantations have occurred more recently. The first transplant of a lower limb was reported only in 2006, when the normal lower limb of a three-month-old conjoined twin, who was not going to survive, was transplanted to her otherwise healthy sister, with the return of muscle function, sensory responses and control. Such incremental developments occur each year.

This pacey chronology captures the mood of heroic medicine. Boosted by advances in anesthesia, surgical technique and cryobiology, surgeons have been able to maintain viable cadaveric tissue and so to speak of the 'shelf life' of different organs. Immunological and pharmacological research led to the successful development of the immunosuppressive drug cyclosporine and then the drug FK506 (Brent 1997), further improving the outcomes of people after transplantation, making organ and tissue transplants routine and encouraging their broad public acceptance. By the early 1990s, successful repeat transplants had occurred, too, precipitating the escalated demand for organs and the increased expectation of such surgery as a way of extending life.

In Australia, these developments had major impact. Australians are reluctant donors and the waiting lists for donor organs are lengthy, leading scientists to revisit questions of the technical compatibility of xenotransplantation and cloning. Embryonic stem cell and cloning legislation was passed at a federal level in 2006. Victorian state legislation in May 2007 furthered research with therapeutic cloning through somatic cell nuclear transfer in mind. The primary brake on these developments has been difficulties in immunocompatibility, not ethics. Since 1963, nearly 46,000 Australians (in a population of 22 million at time of writing) have had organ or tissue transplants. Around 20 percent of people on dialysis – some 2,000 of 10,000 – in any year are awaiting an organ match. In any month, around 1,800 people are on the official (government) organ and tissue transplant registry, waiting for a donor, and about 800 per annum receive a transplant of any kind. Further, in 2010, there were only 309 registered donors, despite considerable institutional promotion to encourage donation, and despite the fact that all Australians can make a living will by annotating their driving license and, in the absence of a living will, a bereaved family can choose to donate tissues or organs. People make rather different decisions about the integrity of the body in life and in death. While Australians are happy to accept tissue and organ transplants compared to Europe and U. S., in contrast they have a very low rate of organ and tissue donation – one of the lowest donation rates in the industrialized world. In this chapter, drawing on accounts from people who have donated or received kidneys, I explore ideas about reciprocity, altruism, embodiment and the constitution of self. These all influence the transplantation economy within this country. Here, the tensions of substance and identity are played out below the surface, but as I illustrate, they ripple to the surface as they impact on social bodies.

A Mechanical Life

Kidney disease is common. Official US estimates are that around 9 percent of the population has chronic kidney disease, although only one in ten of them may be aware of the condition. In Australia, around 7.5 percent have reduced kidney function; one in 400 has end-stage renal disease and requires ongoing treatment.

Kidneys fail for multiple reasons. The most common causes of failure are hypertension, diabetes nephropathy and glomerulonephritis (in which kidney 'filters' become inflamed), but kidney failure occurs also due to infection, congenital diseases such as polycystic kidney disease, physiological anomalies, connective tissue diseases, cancer, and damage from certain anti-inflammatory drugs, lithium and cyclosporine. The growing incidence and absolute number of people with diabetes mellitus and/or cardiovascular disease, too, has led to greater numbers of people with chronic kidney disease, and so an incremental demand for dialysis and potentially for transplant surgery. For most people with end-stage renal disease who have been on dialysis for an extended period, a kidney transplant is the promise of a turning point and an extended life.

While many people who have received or are waiting for a transplant have had a long history of urinary or kidney problems leading to chronic renal failure, for others, kidney failure was unexpected and dramatic. Those on whose narratives I draw reflect this broad spectrum. La Fontaine, for example, had had urinary tract infections from infancy, but she was already 43 when her kidneys began to deteriorate rapidly and her need for a transplant became desperate. Tracy developed polycystic kidney disease in her teens, and by her early 20s had multiple cysts and chronic renal failure. Tatiana was in her 20s with two small children when she became ill. Her doctor felt she was under stress and advised her to rest; a year later, she was diagnosed with kidney function loss and was placed on dialysis. Nathan noticed sudden swelling in his feet after a game of squash; six weeks later he had acute renal failure.

The first step towards a kidney transplant for these and other participants was their need for dialysis, forcing them to deal with "sudden, dramatic change," as Rick described in the epigraph to this chapter: when "your natural life has ended. You rely on machines to keep you alive." Dialysis involves the artificial filtering of blood through a semi-permeable membrane, immersed in a circulating medium of either a purified liquid or solvent. People have a choice of two methods. The first, usually undertaken three times a week for about four hours at a time, is hemodialysis. Prior to commencing this process, a fistula is made usually on the lower arm (sometimes a leg) or, if no vessel is suitable, a thin plastic vascular graft is used to join an artery and vein so that blood can be drained and cleaned. Once connected to the dialysis machine, blood from the large artery flows through a disposable tube to the machine. The blood is kept at body temperature and flows through a semi-permeable tube immersed in constantly changing dialyzing fluid. Waste products and excess water diffuse across the membrane, and clean blood is returned to the body through the vein. In Australia, hemodialysis usually occurs at self-care satellite clinics or in hospital outpatient departments, although people can have home dialysis, enabling the process to occur, without assistance, while they sleep.

The alternative to hemodialysis is peritoneal dialysis, either Continuous Ambulatory Peritoneal Dialysis (CAPD) or Automated Peritoneal Dialysis (APD). In either case, a permanent catheter is inserted into the abdomen to facilitate the flow of fluid into and from the peritoneal cavity. With CAPD, the process is repeated four times a day. The peritoneal membrane is used as a filter so that waste products can be removed, with dialyzing fluid introduced into the peritoneum surrounding the intestines. Four or so hours after the fluid is introduced, the used fluid is drained into a waste bag via a catheter. Since dialyzing fluid is home-delivered in Australia on a monthly basis and the method can be performed anywhere, it offers people some control over their own space, time and mobility. With an alternative peritoneal method, the catheter is attached at night to a machine called a cycler, and six or more exchanges occur while the person sleeps. By day, the solution remains in the body so that dialysis continues to occur.

A person who has had abdominal surgery will be placed on hemodialysis, but usually the choice and location of procedure – hemodialysis or peritoneal dialysis, at home, hospital or satellite center – is elective, with little or no difference in outcomes (Mendelssohn 2004; Kutner, Zhang,

Barnhart, Collins 2005). Globally and in the U. S., around 85 percent of dialysis is hemodialysis, although there are significant differences across cultures. In Australia, less than 80 percent use hemodialysis; in Mexico, it is less than 20 percent. Patient preference is conventionally associated with life style and age, but choice is also influenced by infrastructure, cultural and individual understandings of the processes, perceptions of the relative invasiveness of the two, and local variations in access, cost, level of services, funding mechanisms and support systems.

No-one I interviewed had opted for nocturnal procedures, and the choice, therefore, was either COPD at home or hemodialysis at an outpatient clinic. People who chose hemodialysis did so because of their discomfort at "having a tube in your belly," and because hemodialysis took less time and reduced work disruptions. Most people on hemodialysis, whether or not in paid employment, went to the hospital at the end of day; those with family responsibilities arranged for their children to be fed, bathed and put to bed by their partners or own parents.

As noted, the creation of a fistula, whereby an artery is joined to a vein under the skin, usually near the wrist, to make a larger vessel, is the necessary first step, and is undertaken ideally three to four months before hemodialysis commences so that the walls of the vein are strong enough for dialysis and do not collapse when in use. Tatiana, for example, had a fistula created three months before dialysis was scheduled to commence, with the aim of having the operation while she was 'well' so that she could "bounce back" and have "one less thing to cope with":

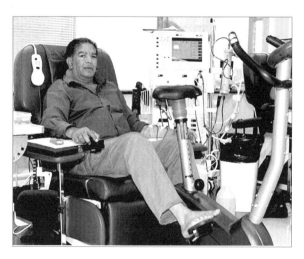

Figure 6.1 Man exercising while receiving haemodialysis treatment. Courtesy of *Renal Society of Australasia Journal.*

It just makes life a little less traumatic, I feel, because after being on dialysis and watching everybody else come in, and having all those feelings of new tablets, new lifestyle, coping with the machine, coping with being at the hospital, that's so much for anybody to cope with, and then you are going to have an operation…. Having a fistula (in advance) is just one less thing to have and I'm glad I had mine done [early].

The fistula appears like a swollen artery or a rope, sensigenous and perceptible. The flow of blood through the fistula creates visible pulsing and a 'buzzy' or 'purring' feeling, causing sleep disturbances for some people because of its noise. Participants often placed a pillow over their arm to mute the sound, but then would take it off for fear of squashing and damaging the fistula. Such protective moves operated in other circumstances, of course; participants were consistently self-conscious of and hypersensitive of risks to their fistula. Rick would often stop in his tracks if he felt a particular physical activity might lead to injury; La Fontaine wore a wrist guard when she played sport to protect her fistula. Most participants were also self-conscious of the appearance of the fistula and wore long sleeve shirts to hide it, they said, as well as to disguise needles marks to avoid people assuming that they were using illicit injectible drugs. Some participants, however, took advantage of the unusualness of the fistula; in the same way that small children were fascinated by artificial legs and stomas, they were fascinated by the 'buzzer' on the arm of a person on dialysis, and with the feel of pulsing blood. Such interactions helped people on dialysis overcome their common sense of social discomfort. One participant had an adult friend, too, who would playfully grab her fistula, joking, "Oh, you always give me a buzz." This was one of the few instances, however, when the fistula slipped from being a source of sensitivity and embarrassment to an item of play.

Hemodialysis requires that the individual is connected to the machine through two needles and tubes, one tube to take blood to the dialysis machine and the second to return dialyzed blood back to the body. Despite assurances from doctors and nurses that the process was pain free, participants found the process often unpleasant and sometimes painful, particularly if they had a 'blow' (venal puncture causing bleeding into tissue). Each visit to the hospital for dialysis potentially could be problematic, and people often felt some suspense about nurses being able to find a vein. Once the ordeal of the insertion of the needle was over, people still would have to wait to get onto a machine, and while undergoing dialysis, to restrict fluid intake.

When you first go in, you just want the needles in. With me, as long as the needles are in and they haven't blown, I don't mind how long I wait until I get on the machine. It's just getting that needle in. Once that needle is in, I'm actually quite relaxed, but then that's really just the start of it, because then you've got four hours and in that time you have to sort of be quite diligent with what you drink and what you eat in between, so you don't have too much fluid to take off. Sometimes they miss and then we have a blow which is like, it puffs up like a little volcano, and it's actually just the blood going into the rest of the tissue and it hurt, it hurts a lot, it's painful to you and you can't use that bit again. So, if you have lots of areas, I have five, then you've got other areas (of the vein) to use and alternate because when you are talking three times a week for three years, it's an awful lot to use the same. (Tatiana)

If I over-drank, you know, had more than my limited amount of water, they had trouble trying to flush out my system. And the machine: that was the scary part because I always think of the worst thing, in case of fire and all that. What do you do if you are hooked up to a machine? You are tied down to a machine and what can you do if something like that happens, everybody running off and you are left with the machine. (Lisa)

Research participants emphasized several points. First, the insertion of the needle could be painful and so caused anxiety, and many people found the needles always unpleasant. If the nurse failed to draw blood or the needle slipped, the resultant 'blow' caused further pain and bruising. Once the tubes were attached, the person must wait to go onto the dialysis machine, and then is 'tied' to the machine for two to four hours. Many found going to a hospital routinely very unpleasant. John, for instance, described hemodialysis as "a horrible way to live."

All respondents also spoke of the difficulty of adhering to dietary restrictions and especially limited fluid intake. Forced to monitor liquids, water became an obsession. People spoke of waking up several times a night for an ice cube, sneaking to the fridge for an extra drink: "It was just terrible because I used to love my water and it was just torture, I couldn't drink it" (Lisa). La Fontaine elaborated on this when she discussed the fine-tuned monitoring and heightened self-surveillance related to fluid intake and excretion, drawing on the technical explanations provided to her to explain her decision to retain one partially-functioning kidney:

What I had to consider was that with the fluid intake, you could have 500 mls [a little less than one pint], plus whatever you were passing. Now, I was still passing 400 mls, so that meant a lot to me. That meant I could have 900 mls of fluid. As you know one cup of rice is 100 mls, one medium sized tomato is 100 mls. It [the fluid] was all in food. And me that loves water – water is my favorite drink – that was very difficult. So if I'd had both kidneys out, I'd be down to 500 mls a day and my quality of life, once again, would go down. That's why, in the end, I chose to keep the right one [kidney], even though there wasn't much there, and have that 400 mls. With the fluid, I was very careful. If you didn't have to take off too much fluid when you had dialysis, you didn't feel as washed out.

With hemodialysis, the functions of the body are externalized. Blood flows out of the body, via the needles and tubes, through the dialysis machine; the blood is 'washed' outside of the body. In contrast, with CAPD, matter is fed into the body – the dialyzing liquid runs into the peritoneum via the catheter – and the process is internal; the 'washing' of blood takes place in the peritoneum. People who were uncomfortable with hemodialysis because of the needles, or who found attending hospital disturbing, felt that CAPD gave them personal independence, while also preserving whatever kidney function they had left. CAPD was also seen as less invasive despite the routine daily interruptions, the emphasis on local hygiene and the risk of peritonitis. Dave, for example, found training for CAPD relatively easy and learned quickly to adapt and improvise:

> I was at home within the week doing dialysis on my own and I was discovering that it didn't restrict me, given that they can deliver your dialysis stuff anywhere in the world. So going interstate to visit my parents was not a hassle; I'd do my dialysis in the car, heating up the bag by leaving it on the dashboard to warm in the sun while driving, and then putting the bag on the roof of the car to do the dialysis. I was determined not to let it restrict my life at all. If a motel didn't have a microwave, I'd heat the bag by running it under the hot tap in the sink. If that's what you've got to do, you do it. You improvise, you find ways, and as long as you maintain your hygienic techniques of doing things, there's no problem.

The Ultimate Gift

In Australia, people requiring hemodialysis can arrange to call in at any hospital if traveling, and as Dave recounts above, people on CAPD can carry supplies of dialyzing fluid and collect additional supplies as required when on the road. People can stay on dialysis for years. The underlying pathology may shape decisions relating to the ongoing management of renal failure, and people may need to move from peritoneal to hemodialysis, then to transplant, for the best chances of survival and quality of life. But in any case, few people aspire to remain on dialysis by choice, because of routine machine dependency and the constant surveillance of the body. Kidney transplantation appears the "light at the end of the tunnel" (Rick); it is cost-efficient and offers a longer life span and better quality of life. But organ supply is short globally and in particular settings, including Australia, as discussed above. Australians on dialysis and hoping for a cadaver organ may have to wait six or more years until a match between organ donor and recipient. Not all live this long.

Transplantation surgery does not eliminate interaction with medicine. The reverse is the case; surveillance and medication are ongoing. Even so, donor recipients are acutely aware of the truth of the trope of 'gift of life.' Donation requests in particular play on the metaphor of 'gift.' The organ itself, its gift by a living donor or the family of a person who is deceased, and the surgical procedure are all characterized as 'gifts of life' both by those who have had transplants (see below) and by consumer groups, medical organizations and government agencies seeking to encourage donation.

In 2006, the Australian federal government organized a National Competition for Organ and Tissue Donation for secondary and higher education students with three streams: the design of a *Flame of Life* device for use as the national symbol for organ and tissue donation, the design of a poster to encourage donation ("1 organ and tissue donor can save up to 10 people"), and, for secondary school students, a poem about organ and tissue donation ("Life, enhanced/ Thanks to a stranger") (Australia 2006). In 2007 again, the government invited secondary and higher education students to enter a national art and poetry competition to "portray the gift of organ and tissue donation in a positive and effective way." As the announcement on the departmental website explained, "entering the competition is a gift in itself, by raising awareness among entrants and their peers about the vital need for organ and tissue transplants and donations" (Australia 2007). The prizes, awarded on World Day for Organ Donation and Transplantation (October 26, 2007) and unveiled at the national media launch of Australian Organ Donor Awareness Week in February 2008, were to be awarded to both students and their schools, encouraging institutional support for the competition. Similarly, the government website of the Organ and Tissue Authority Advisory Council, DonateLife (www.donatelife.gov.au), and other websites of national organizations involved in organ and tissue donation and transplantation, including independent donation agencies and banks, community groups and individuals working to increase donations, all use the rhetoric of the gift in personal testimonies in different media and in everyday discourse.

Fox and Swazey (1992:33) and Lock (2001) have argued convincingly that organ donation cannot be isolated to the people involved, that is, the donor and recipient. They note, as did Simmons (1971) two decades earlier, that the shortfall of supply to demand and the immunological advantages of live-related donors have both led to 'inner and outer' pressures from physicians and other family members on individuals to be donors to kin. Indeed, the Australians Donate website cautions that this reflects that "donation is the one form of generosity that can't be spontaneous; it depends on potential donors registering their consent and discussing it with their families, friends and partners" (Australians Donate: The Peak National Body for Organ and Tissue Donation for Transplantation 2007). Despite the rhetoric of the gift, therefore, unconditional giving is uncommon, particularly in the event of live donations. This is hardly surprising for anthropologists familiar with Mauss's work (1967). Gifts are a way of sustaining social relations, within families and between individuals or groups linked instrumentally and emotionally. Normatively, gifts are exchanged; the paradox in organ and tissue donation is its one-way flow. Giving a cornea, pancreas, lung or a kidney, through a living will or in life, is therefore a supreme example of altruism. The gift cannot be returned in kind or in equivalence, either to the donor or the donor's family. Further, the gift is entrusted to the recipient in ways over which neither giver nor receiver has control: organs can be rejected, and may have to be removed. The live donor, too, must undergo surgery more extensive than that required by the recipient; all study participants spoke of this as an added cost taken into consideration by the donor and other family members. For the donor, too, there is always the possibility of damage to the remaining kidney. At the same time, as Fox and Swazey note, the symbolic meaning implicated in organ donation – to save someone's life – "virtually obliges every family member at least to consider making such a gift" (33).

In practice, the extent to which families discuss possible donation varies, as does the communication of this to the potential recipient, and so the outcomes of such decision-making also vary. Receiving a kidney or making a live donation are not easy decisions, and raise for those involved questions of reciprocity, altruism, embodiment, and the nature of self. Giving was problematic for some of my participants, but so, too, was acceptance of the gift. A recipient may not wish a live donor to undergo extensive surgery, pain and possible lengthy hospitalization and convalescence, nor wish to take on the risk that live donation entails; he or she may feel that receipt of an organ from a living relative will complicate the relationship and create a debt impossible to repay.

The decision to donate was immediate and unwavering only in one case in my study; for Liz, who donated a kidney to her son Nathan. Yet even in this case, Liz made the decision not spontaneously, but in response to a doctor's intimation that it would be "a lot better" for Nathan were he to have a transplant rather than remain on dialysis. Her theoretical refusal to be a donor was positioned morally, therefore, as passive homicide, or at the very least, the instantiation of 'being a bad mother.' Liz's offer to donate, even so, was initially rejected because she smoked, and consequently her older son, Glen, volunteered. But as Liz told the story, Glen "has always had a yellow streak, pretty wide" (i.e., he was a coward), and he withdrew his offer when he found out what the surgery would entail. Since Liz was compatible histologically, she commenced a determined fitness regime: she gave up smoking, she moved to live independently from her partner who still smoked, and she exercised, motivated as much by the medical report that described her as "a tad overweight" as she was by the impediment of her smoking to her possible involvement as a donor.

While the primary criterion to be a live donor is immunological compatibility, other social, medical and family factors influence decisions, as Liz's example illustrates. In various respects, doctors, family members and the person in need of a transplant balance these factors in terms of present and future. Does the person on dialysis really need a new kidney now, such that a living donor is essential? Would the potential donor's health be compromised by surgery now, or in the future? Do the benefits of transplantation outweigh the health risks for the donor?

The decision-making that lead to Carol's donation illustrates how these various risks are weighed. Carol's family considered her to be the

most suitable donor for her sister Sheila for social not medical reasons: she
was not married and did not have children. While others in the family had
"sort of thought, well, if this had to be done then they would do it as well,"
Sheila rejected several people as possible donors: "Why should it be dad?
After all, he's got our family, he works so hard, he looks after all of us. What
if something happened to him?" Sheila's mother was willing to be a donor,
but Sheila rejected her, too, because she felt that she was "too old." While
Sheila stressed that she didn't want anyone in the family to feel obliged to
donate, she, her parents and other siblings all saw Carol as the obvious and
ideal donor. Carol reflected:

> I'm sure secretly she did hope that somebody would [donate]. She
> said, "You don't have to do this, you know," and I said, "I know." She
> said, "Look, I'll be forever grateful," and I said, "Well, I don't expect
> you to be grateful either." I don't expect her for the rest of her days to
> drop everything and say, "What do you want me to do for you?" I just
> don't think it works that way; I don't think it can.

Carol was the ideal donor from her family's perspective, because they
considered her to have no family of her own. Her life-partner Jeanne did
not agree, but Carol thought that this reflected Jeanne's anxiety, insecu-
rity and the fragile relationship she had with Carol's family, and this was
not a compelling reason for Carol to withdraw her offer to donate. Carol
said that she felt "very confident through the whole process.... I wasn't
waking up in the middle of the night or lying awake thinking some dreadful things will happen to me, I really did feel very confident." She felt this
confidence helped Jeanne also.

This family-referenced decision-making – who has the least to lose,
who is the fittest – reflected the considerations of most respondents and
their families. Those who became recipients spent long hours weighing
up the risks and benefits of accepting donor offers. As Dave pointed out,
it's "morally a big question for people because they [donors] do have to go
on living with only one kidney." Tatiana, for example, rejected her sister's
offer of a kidney because of her concern about her long term health and her
possible future: "I was worried that it was a family, hereditary thing, and
she hadn't married or had children. I don't think I could live with myself
if her other kidney failed." John's father had initially offered to donate a
kidney ten years before surgery, and John had resisted because he wasn't
willing to put his father's life at risk. John subsequently had two unsuccessful cadaver organ transplants; following the second rejection, the

renal consultant suggested that John have a live-related transplant. Both his parents and sister offered, both parents proved compatible, and his father insisted that it be he.

Lisa originally rejected her brother's offer, too; she was determined to 'fight' the disease herself. When her condition deteriorated and problems with dialysis developed, her doctor suggested that she accept his offer. Her sisters were both married, and her older brother frequently traveled, was away at the time that transplantation was being discussed, and so was not available for tests. Her brother Gerry was "youngest and single and healthy" and so best suited prima facie to be a donor. Lisa felt guilty initially when she was asked to reconsider his offer, because she didn't want him to have surgery, but when she approached him and asked him directly, there was no problem: "He said, 'Yeah, I'll do it.' He was just like that, 'Just tell me what I have to do.' There was no 'If I do this, you have to do that.'" As she explained, however, his response was not sufficient, and the operation was cancelled because the psychiatrist felt that Gerry was not ready:

> I was a bit upset then because you know, you have yourself psyched up and everything. I knew Gerry was fine; he'd gone through all the tests and everything. We'd both seen the psychiatrist and I thought everything was fine.... Nobody would tell me why [the operation was cancelled]. Later on, I found out that it was the psychiatrist who felt that Gerry wasn't ready. I thought, how did he make that assumption? How did he come to that conclusion because we both went and saw him, we saw him individually, there was no pressure on Gerry. I said he [Gerry] could back out any time. So, there was no pressure. Like, he was willing to do it for me and he was ready as well, and I couldn't understand how somebody else could think for him, that he wasn't ready.

Family members all find it difficult to decide to donate, but it is even more difficult when there is resistance from people to assess their suitability as a possible donor or resistance to donating. Terry, for example, was originally unwilling to donate a kidney to his son Brett, who needed a kidney transplant after he had surgery for peritonitis. Terry, his wife and eldest son were all tested for compatibility. Subsequent tests indicated that there would be surgical complications were his wife to donate, and so the 'decision' as put to the family by the consultant surgeon was for Terry to donate. But Terry had not thought through the implications of surgery and donation, and he was reluctant:

Initially I said no, and I think that was because it is a protective thing for yourself. You think about it: I was given these [kidneys] to support my life, you know, and I'm going to compromise that. But then you go further into the implications of that. It came down to giving Brett quality of life. The "no, I'm not" was an initial thing. It is like someone putting a question to you: "Will you do this?" without giving you … well, there is no way you can sort of break into that gently. Once we'd gone into it all and realized how things were, it wasn't really a difficult choice.

Accounts such as Terry's illustrate the stress placed on family members and the inherent tensions that this exposes. Earlier, I noted that Liz regarded her older son to be a coward when he refused to donate to his brother. Tracy's account again illustrates how decisions concerning donation expose fissures in family relationships. Tracy's mother could not donate because, like Tracy, she had polycystic kidney disease. Tracy's siblings did not offer to be tested for compatibility, and her father was never able to overcome his own sense of fear:

Dad went off and found out what blood type he was and saw his doctor about donating his kidney. He got all the details about it and went away, and got very, very scared. He was going to keep it under wraps and not saying anything to me and just think about it, and then maybe come and talk to me. Unfortunately, Mum said something to me, and then I'm thinking, "Oh wow, this is great, I'm getting a kidney, this could be happening, I don't know if I want it, but gee whiz, the thought is nice." And then my dad knocks on the door one day, and says, "Look, you know, I've thought about it and I really can't do it because it scares me too much, but if you really need it and you're desperate for it, like you're dying, I'll give it to you." I think he had to tell me this because Mum had told me. I was … I wanted him to come up to me and say, "Sweetheart, I love you so much, you're my daughter, I want to give you a kidney." Then I would have turned around and said, "No thanks, Dad, that's fine," because I didn't want to put him through it. But I still wanted him to make the offer … all I wanted was the offer, but he never did, and I was angry.

The emotional and symbolic weight of the gift is clear. Tracy saw the gesture as the gift; in talking to me, she insisted that she would not have accepted it while there was a possibility of cadaver organ donation. But she felt deeply rejected by her father through his failure to make the gesture – the offer of donation. At other times in conversation, Tracy spoke of her parents' coldness towards her, their reluctance to hold her or to provide her with a warm and supportive relationship. She saw her father's inability to donate a kidney as evidence of his inability to express his love for her, and she questioned the veracity of such emotion entirely.

My final example of a live-related donation echoes the theme of altruism. Rosie was Rick's niece (his sister's daughter). For several reasons, including their relational distance and because she lived in another city, she was not in close communication with Rick or other family members, and so there was no social pressure on her to donate. As Rick tells the story, he was "never ever what you'd call close with her.... I'd probably see her once every two years or so for a wedding or something like that." Rosie learned of her uncle's rapid deterioration of health during a telephone conversation with her mother, and without Rick knowing, she found out his blood type and checked on what was involved with donation. At a family wedding, she came up to him, and as he described it:

> She said, "Uncle Rick, I'm going to give you my kidney," and that blew me away. I went to pieces. I sat there. In fact, I'm getting a little bit thingy [weepy] about it now. I was in total shock. I didn't know what to say. It took a couple of weeks, with us communicating by phone because of her living [in another state]. As I say, I only see her once every so often, and she is still a young woman; she is 35 years of age, she is married, she has got two children. I thought to myself – look, you know, you just don't come up and say that sort of thing. I was never ever what you'd call close with her. So for her to have done that, really, to me it is just something special.

Here, the strengths of kinship and generosity of spirit outweighed the moral obligations of gift-exchange, although Rick was conscious of these and spent much time working through these questions. Supported by her husband, children and mother, Rosie had a full medical work-up. Rick had long conversations with Rosie and her husband prior to the operation, on the phone and face-to-face, including confirming that her husband was comfortable about her decision. Rosie and her husband both had psychiatric counseling. Rick was initially cautious, worried that the offer might not follow through and then gaining confidence: "I was very, very positive, but always, you know, expecting at any stage that she might change her mind or whatever. But I started to see that it was going to happen; things would happen, sort of thing." Rick understood Rosie's motivation as deriving from two sources. She had a friend who had donated a kidney, and consequently she had personal exposure to and an understanding of end-stage renal disease, dialysis and transplantation that was very different from that gleaned from booklets, brochures and the advice of medical personnel. Rick also attributed the ideology and everyday interactions of her family as informing her action; he regarded her family, those of his older sister and her children, as "so close and so supportive of each other … they are pretty much spread around Australia, but if something goes wrong they are all there helping out." From Rick's and Rosie's standpoint, in the end, giving a kidney was simply an obvious way of 'helping out.'

Others, too, came to understand that the gift of a kidney from a parent was a part of parenting, a demonstration of parental love, and a dimension of a moral economy of kinship. John, who for years refused to accept a kidney from his father, now reflected that he would do the same thing: "If I had a child, I'd have no right to deny him and I would give him that gift and I have a right to do as much as I possibly can. So that is how I came to terms with it and I have absolutely no problems at all with that." This, of course, is why Tracy was so hurt; her father had made explicit his inability to offer what she considered to be the ultimate expression of unconditional love.

On a Cloud of Grief

Accounts of the decision-making to donate and the subsequent surgery capture the awful excitement of this period: delays while a living donor undergoes histological and psychiatric assessment, or while the potential recipient waits for advice of a match, then waiting to assess the success or failure of the transplant. The donor and recipient involved in live-related transplants spend much time preparing for surgery, with medical and surgical consultants and psychiatrists ensuring that both are of sound mind, and that other family members are equally comfortable with the decision and fully appreciate its risks. As Lisa illustrated of her own experience, at any point, the surgeon or psychiatrist might stall the process. Liz and Nathan also had a 'false start,' with Liz's weight and smoking both contraindicating surgery. The waiting was frustrating in both cases, but the outcome was able to be manipulated if not certain, and the timelines relatively easy to predict. In contrast, those requiring cadaver organs wait for the morally unacceptable – someone else's death. Since a 'healthy kidney' is usually in a healthy body, the donor is most likely to have died by trauma, often in a vehicular accident, or from an aneurysm or stroke. Cadaveric organs are matched as quickly as possible for histocompatibility including ABO blood typing, and checked for cytotoxic antibodies, although the presence of viruses such as cytomegalavirus is not regarded as contraindicative.

The likelihood that the donor was a young healthy person who had been killed in a motor accident or otherwise had died suddenly is high, so much so that Tracy's mother searched for publicly available clues to the identity of the donor. She purchased and scrutinized all the newspapers she could get while Tracy was in the hospital, and persistently pressed her daughter about whether she had heard a helicopter before surgery, a possible clue to an out-of-town death and the delivery of harvested tissue and organs.

A sudden death, tests for compatibility, advice to the potential recipient and subsequent surgery all take place in a matter of hours, and consequently, while recipients from living donors spoke of the drawn out process, those who received cadaveric organs couched transplantation surgery in terms of high drama and excitement. Dave, for example, was interviewed a little over a year after he had had a kidney transplant, but he gave a detailed account of his transplant surgery with a sense of immediacy and attention to detail that made it seem only weeks earlier. On a particular day, at 12:30 p.m., Dave received a phone call from his surgeon, advising him of a kidney match. He had prepared a list for action in the event of a transplant, and he adhered to it faithfully: "Make a flight booking, organize transport to airport, advise people that you're going to hospital, pack clothes for ten days, and so on." One hour later Dave was boarding the plane, mindful that the longer the delay, the greater the risk of deterioration of the kidney and hence the risk of rejection. In the taxi to the hospital, Dave turned on his mobile phone:

> There were about twenty messages – people ringing up [saying] "someone's just told me you've got a kidney!" and everyone's trying to ring you not realizing that it might be really important to keep the phone line free. I hadn't been able to contact my parents. I gave my mum my old mobile phone in case we might need it for this, and the one day I needed to bloody well contact her on her mobile phone, she's got the darn thing turned off and she wasn't at home. So I was frantically leaving messages with all my mum's friends, saying "Can you please let my parents know I've got a kidney, I'm on my way to the hospital!" The cab driver must have been listening to me, and heard me mention the words "transplant" and "on my way to the hospital right now" and suddenly he found that there was lead in his foot [i.e., he

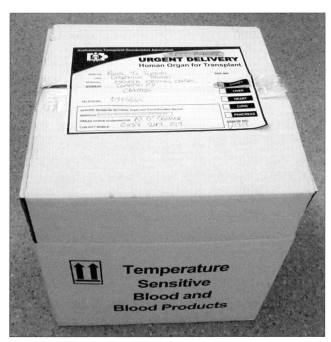

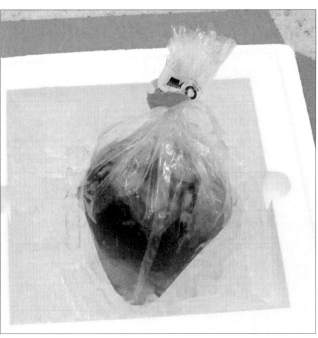

Figure 6.2
Kidney for
Transplant.
Photographs
by the author.

drove faster]. [People] might know nothing about organ transplantation, but there's just like this collective assumption that it's something
that's really urgent and it has to happen quickly and it's battle stations.
So I was very appreciative of that.

While cadaver organ transplants avoid potentially complicated
kinship links, the affiliation and sense of indebtedness transfers to an
anonymous family. As Dave put it, the organ is "brought in on a cloud of
grief" of people unknown. People who had received cadaveric transplants
spoke of having prayed for a kidney, and were now shocked by their own
self-centeredness that they might have wished someone else to die so that
they might live. Those who had transplants under such circumstances
experienced confused sensations of grief and gratitude. Tracy was overwhelmed by the paradox of a life for a death:

> Someone had to die for me to get this kidney.... Because of them,
> somebody I've never met before, it's the most incredible feeling.... I
> had a day when I sobbed and sobbed for the family who lost whoever,
> their child or whoever, or the wife who had lost her husband, I've got a
> fair idea that it [the kidney] was from a male. I had to go through a day
> of grieving for that family. I just sobbed and sobbed, and felt so sorry
> for them. It's so wonderful that they gave me this gift.

The usual means by which transplant social workers encourage recipients to manage this sense of grief is by letter writing. Recipients or family
members write to the family of the donor; if the letter is not returned,
the recipient knows that the letter has been received and accepted. Not
all families who agree to organ donation want this communication, however, even anonymously. And those who wrote to bereft families described
doing so as "the hardest thing I've ever had to do," finding it almost impossible to put on paper how they felt, yet are driven to do so by an imperative
to communicate their thanks to the bereaved family. Dave gave a brief
speech and read a poem at an annual church service for organ donor
families and recipients. La Fontaine was inspired to write a letter before a
church service for donors and their families was held:

> I just thought what to say, [that] I can never really imagine what you're
> going through but to a certain extent I know what it's like to lose
> someone ... I was trying to say that I could relate to a certain degree
> and then I just – I can't think what else I said, but I said, I just can't
> tell you how much this has changed my life and what it was like, and
> you will always be in my thoughts and my prayers, your lost one and

yourselves. I still pray for them – not every night, but whenever I think of it – and nearly every day I say, thank you, Lord. Now, I would like to write another letter – I should write another letter to them because I often think of them.

Jemima also reflected on the impossibility of offering solace to someone she will never know, but who she thinks about constantly. In her case, her mother was the letter writer:

You know, my mother has actually written a letter, but she has never posted it, and she rang to see how she goes about sending it. I just feel I wouldn't know what to say. Thank you seems so inadequate. What do you say? Their child, their husband, whatever, their relative has died, you know; you feel so inadequate saying anything, but this particularly. I just wouldn't know what to say to them.

Others found it impossible to write but fantasized meeting the family and embracing them:

Like, I think I would rather meet them than put it down in a letter.... I didn't want to know, but if I happened to meet them, parents who lost their 20-year-old son in a car accident; if I met them, it would be the most incredible experience because I could give them a hug. But I'm not going to and there's no use dreaming about it or thinking about it. (Tracy)

Part of me would like to know who it was; part of me does not. Like, I think I would rather meet them than put it down in a letter.... Nothing is going to bring that person back. Somebody has died tragically. (Jemima)

Jemima and Tracy capture the paradox of being alive because someone else has died – what Dave refers to as "tangible bitter-sweetness" – and their ambivalence about knowing the family and the circumstances of the donor's death. Several participants expressed the hope that the donor was not a child. Most assumed that it was a young adult, consistent with stereotypes of general good health and fitness, and of a life cut short by a motor accident. Dave most articulately elaborated on the curiosity of meeting and thanking the family in person, while dismissing absolutely the importance of the personal history of the donor – the prehistory of his new kidney:

I got my life back. I think it's horrible that they lost their life. It's tragic that they lost their life, but it wasn't for nothing. In a sense, I feel a kind of obligation to look after myself, to give this donated kidney the best chance possible…. Every day that I wake up and last another day is, in a sense, a memorial to that person because it's almost like their life continuing through another person. Meeting the family would not be about who the donor was. It's deeper than that, it's deeper than gender, deeper than background, deeper than income, family size, where they lived; it's just the fact that another human being saw, somewhere inside themselves, that this [donating] was a good thing to do. And I don't care who they were, that doesn't matter to me, it's just fantastic what they did and I would just like to think that that person's family has a sense of that … that this was a bloody fantastic thing to do. It doesn't need any more than that. They did something that was really good, probably the greatest thing you could ever do.

Tatiana was an exception to the cadaveric and live-related transplants described in this chapter. She was the recipient of an anonymous live donor. Initially, her surgeon told her simply that it was "not *actually* a cadaver kidney." Her response was a practical one related to whether the surgery would proceed – "I'm going, what's wrong? The kidney is there. I've got to be there, I've got to get it done." She only learned of the circumstances of the donation much later. She reflected on the donation and the healthiness of the kidney:

I assume it [the donor] was somebody who was possibly a little bit older than me. I don't know why, don't ask me that, I don't know why, I just guess. I assume it's a male because I don't think a woman would…. With what I know, what happened, they didn't want the kidney, they just believed there was pain in there, in that area, and they believed they needed it out badly and the doctor said there was nothing wrong with the kidney at all and they were like, there's something wrong. I don't think that's a woman. I just can't … no. I look at it [the kidney] like a stray. Nobody wanted it and now it's got a home and it's well loved and it's thriving and doing really well…. When I found out the circumstances, that they didn't want the kidney, they just wanted it out of the body, I thought, "Well, they didn't want it and they didn't care who had it. They didn't care. They just wanted it thrown away or out, that's it, they didn't want it, they didn't care," and I thought, "Oh well, they are okay, I can stop praying. I can just start saying thank you now." I could not imagine that it took one doctor's opinion because that would be, like, not a very good thing. I would be worried if I was the doctor. I would be getting triple, four, five checks to see that I was not the only one. But they said there was nothing wrong with the kidney, and there is nothing wrong with it. It flushed straight away, it came through.

Non-directed kidney donation is very uncommon, but can occur in a number of states in Australia, subject to psychological assessment of the donor, including their motivation and assurance of the lack of financial or other incentives other than personal costs paid by the institution where the transplant is being performed. In many respects, non-directed live organ donation is the ultimate altruistic act; definitionally, it is the gift of a living donor "to help an unknown individual in need" (Transplant Society of Australia and New Zealand 2003). Tatiana speculates that her donor was a man – indeed, she could not imagine a woman would give away a kidney like a "stray" (kitten). As already described, a number of recipients of cadaver organs also speculated on the circumstances of death and the age and sex of the donor. A number reflected, too, on the (im)possibility of meeting the family of the donor. La Fontaine went further; she imagined the physical presence of the donor at a thanksgiving service for donors:

> I started to meditate and as soon as I started to meditate, straightaway there's this face there and straightaway I thought, that's my donor, that's the donor of this kidney. And I got scared, because I thought, I'm never, ever going to – it was just like a hologram – and there was this incredible sadness shown on his face. He was just looking at me, looking incredibly sad, a young man, probably late 20s. I can see his face now. It was just like a hologram. That's now a part of me, and I was trying to get used to someone else being a part of me, and I thought, I'm never going to be alone again ever. I thought, I'll never be able to meditate, there's always going to be someone there; I was scared. So I stopped meditating … I don't know if that person in the meditation was actually the person or was just a person representing someone. But the next night I tried to meditate – I invited them back and said, I'm really sorry, you're welcome, you're naturally welcome in my meditations. But he never came back. I don't know if it really was that person or some figment of my imagination, telling me what to write in the letter. I felt mainly sadness for all his family. Perhaps he was help-ing me write the letter to help his family; I hope it's helping someone. That's my interpretation of it, I could be completely wrong. But I just wrote the letter, sent it the next day, and I felt that it was right. I can still see the face when I think of it. But whenever I think of the donor,

I try not to think of that in case it isn't. I just think of the family donating …but if I think of the donor, yes, I think of that face. I think of it as
a younger man with this face.

La Fontaine's image of the donor of the kidney was corporeal, even
though she reflected that the vision was symbolic – "a person representing someone." She did not take literally, therefore, the association between
the donated organ and its imagined biological owner. Others had more
literal ideas about affiliation. Angelus, for example, extended the notion of
blood ties to include kinship through surgery: "The thing is, you gain new
family with a transplant. So I'd like to meet the family. I don't know why
they don't want to meet me. They're related to me, aren't they? You'd think
they'd want to get to know me." Other respondents had less a sense of kinship, but did have a sense of embodied consciousness of their kidneys.

None was especially disturbed about having a foreign body part.[1] Even
so, Tracy reflected that on a couple of occasions, she had felt that "someone
else" was inside her, and "it's a real, oh, that's a real funny weird sensation
sort of feeling, but it's not been a thing in my mind to want to think about
it." She explained that her hyperawareness of the transplant kidney and its
genesis related to her constant awareness that "it [the kidney] is just under
the skin. I suppose it would be harder for some people who can't feel their
kidneys, but I can actually feel mine. It's a constant reminder." Others
spoke of the 'personality' of their new kidney; they explained changes in
taste and behavior that occurred as their bodies integrated a foreign organ
with its own history. La Fontaine reflected on her change of tastes: "I don't
like whiskey any more. I used to love cold malt whiskey." She rationalized this as the outcome of changes in diet from dialysis, when all she was
ever able to drink, because of restrictions on fluid intake, was straight malt
whiskey with lots of ice cubes. Yet as she notes: "You do change your habits
because of your years on dialysis, you change your habits anyway. But yes,
I often think about, wonder what he was like." Others also refer jokingly
to changes in drinking habits. Terry, for instance, reported that his son
"often jokes about it, I still joke about it. One of the things he says now is
that he never liked beer, but he tells me now that it was my kidneys that
made him like the odd beer or two now. Things like that we joke about, but
nobody thinks that I owe you something because of this."

Terry's comment draws attention, too, to how kin use humor to dilute
any residual tension. Gerry asked his sister Lisa, to whom he had donated
a kidney, to take a photograph of his scar, and told her she'd got the better

kidney. He reassured her that, "As long as I don't go horse riding or motor-bike riding," he would be alright. At the same time, Lisa reflected both that he was well and that she always asked him to look after himself. Gerry still spoke to Lisa, long after surgery, of *his* kidney, the history of the transplant revisited in their everyday conversations. Similarly, Liz worried that her kidney wouldn't "last the distance" for her son, Nathan: "My biggest concern is what happens when my kidney packs in, where do we go from here? He has had several biopsies on my kidney. Every time you get sick, it loses a little bit more of its oomph." Liz cautioned Nathan: "Look, don't try and hang on to that kidney just because ... throw it in the garbage, get rid of it and let's hope for another scenario."

Gendered Bodies

The idea of a kidney as a 'thing,' a device to be thrown in the garbage if it fails to work, is not common. For the most part, research participants tied the organ to its prehistory and speculated on the person's life and on the idea of consubstantiation. According to this logic, a series of assumptions may be made: that the character of a person (personality, ideas, values, tastes and memory) is embedded in the substance of his or her physical body, giving rise to the controversial idea of 'cellular memories' of experiences, personality traits and tastes, that is, that the substance of the whole coexists with the substance of the part. As examined in a UK television documentary *Transplanting Memories* (Krawczyk 2004), the heart was presented as an organ with cellular memory and so the inheritability of personality and preferences. In this study, the kidneys, too, were attributed with the capacity for memory. A number of recipients attributed changes in personality and taste to their 'inheritance,' and took these as clues to the donor's gender. Cadaver organ recipients routinely reflected on the meanings of physical and emotional changes in these terms. While not all recipients ascribed gender to the donor, a number of women assumed that the donor was male, slightly younger than them. This fits with the stereotype of a person who, after a road traffic accident, could be a donor. But men tended to assume that the donor of their kidney was female. Angelus, for example, spoke of the young woman who he imagined to be his donor, for she had brought out the 'feminine side' of him: he believed he had become softer, kinder and more sensitive since his transplant surgery. Several men attributed heightened emotionality post-transplant to having a woman's kidney, although those who had received a kidney from a living-related donor were most likely to be tearful. Women, on the other hand, were more likely to weep when they spoke about their childbearing after transplantation: a new kidney gave them the opportunity of reproduction that other women took for granted.

On the other hand, women sometimes interpreted the masculinizing effects of steroids as evidence of male identity of the cadaveric donor, even though both women and men had sophisticated understandings of the side effects of drugs and consequent bodily change. Prednisolone affected women's libido and temperament, and caused hirsuteness and weight gain. Women said they were more likely after surgery to lose their temper, need to shave and want sex. These side effects did not create the same gendered esthetic problems for men, although hirsuteness caused them some embarrassment related to having to shave twice daily, and some commented on the length of their body hair "as being disconcerting to say the least" (Angelus). Women found the side effects more disturbing as they developed hairs "where they never were before:"

> You get extremely hairy, very, very hairy and that's hard to take, and your hair goes darker. My hair is extremely dark and bushy. I thought to myself, that's easy. I'll just go and get it waxed. But it's not that easy; it needs to be a certain length to actually get it off. I don't think I could last that long. You think everybody is staring at it when they're not really. It's difficult because I have got it all on my ears which I've never had, like there's heaps up here [on her forehead]. A disconcerting thing is that there is this notion of what a female face looks like, and yes, it's that sort of self-consciousness of having facial hair. (Tatiana)

> I have had everything waxed you can think of. I've had my ears waxed. I just, oh my god, because I looked like a hairy gorilla in the beginning. What I did, I had it all waxed and since then, since the drugs were reduced, I've only had to worry about my chin and my ears. I do have hairy arms, but it's not that noticeable. But it's all over my bottom and my back. It bothered me at first. It still bothers me. In fact, I haven't had a sex life. I'm not interested in getting into a relationship. I'm thinking, if I go out with someone and if I end up eventually one day having a relationship, should I go and get all my back and bottom waxed or should I just leave it as it is and have a hairy bottom? (La Fontaine)

La Fontaine's wariness of committing to a new relationship is not simply a matter of her hirsuteness, but of the entwined history of a deteriorating relationship concurrent with her need for dialysis and transplant surgery. Even so, changes in the distribution, quality, thickness and rapidity of growth of hair are an undesirable embodied reminder of the drugs now necessary to prevent rejection of the transplant and to maintain life. Other changes to the body caused greater concern. Changes in weight and the characteristic development of a 'moon face' (Cushingoid features) were common, and often occurred rapidly. People spoke of 'all of a sudden' looking different. Tracy and Tatiana both recalled occasions when people they knew well did not recognize them in the street. Rick mentioned that acquaintances often "had to look pretty hard" to recognize him, and a number of colleagues "had a bit of a problem with it, all the people at work and that sort of thing, people you hadn't seen for a little while, they recognized it [weight gain] straight away, you know, a big change." Tracy recalls the effects on her self-image and self-esteem of having acne, a moon face, and weight gain: "I wouldn't look in the mirror. I just couldn't bear my body. I said to Mum, 'I don't want to see anybody, I don't want to hear from anybody.' I was so odd looking … I was very self-conscious about it."

Several respondents also reflected on changes to libido, mood and wellbeing, although generalization is problematic given differences in their age, sex and time since surgery. Some had a difficult period of recovery and rehabilitation as they battled with organ rejection, nosocomial infections and adverse events. Others reported almost immediately feeling euphoric and energetic after transplant surgery, and maintained that their sex life was better than ever. Given their poor health before surgery and often for years previously, this was hardly surprising, and several who had not had partners at the time of surgery became involved in new relationships. Dave, who was 33, explained how his history of illness and his negative body image (as undesirably fat) shaped his imagined life trajectory, influencing his readiness to establish a romantic/sexual relationship:

> I hadn't been in a relationship for nearly five years, partly through choice because of the whole thing of thinking "no-one would be interested in me anyway," and not being confident enough that somebody could be interested in me just because they are. That whole feeling of "Why would anybody be interested in me?" is almost ludicrous now that I'm in a relationship. It's been a real slap in the face to me. How could I be so fickle to believe that people are only attracted to other people physically anyway? It does go a lot deeper than that and it actually doesn't matter and it's quite amazing to be in a relationship with somebody who doesn't – how can I put this? – accept all of this stuff as

part of who I am, without it being the reason for being with me. That's what I was always worried about – my sympathy value – and that is just so not the case.

These accounts are balanced by reports of unsatisfactory and non-existent sex-lives, shaped by individual illness histories, age and partner status at the time of the transplant. Lisa, for example, was diagnosed with acute renal disease when she was 23 years old. She called off her wedding, although she continued to live with her partner.

No sex. That's something we don't really – well, we do discuss it every now and then, we joke about it, but we are both happy, because like, when I was sick that would be the last thing I would be thinking of because I was just trying to survive, and I don't think he would pressure me into anything. When I was sick we never discussed it. We were just enjoying each other's company, sort of thing, like doing the things we want to do like we were doing before, so we would try and

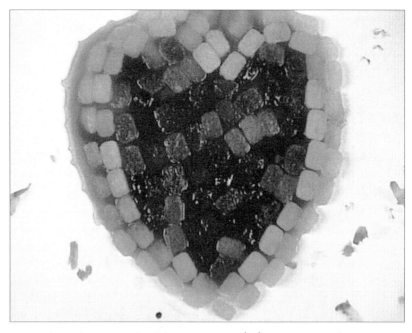

Figure 6.3 Julie Rrap, *Blood & Urine Heart (11)*; 1999. From the Porous Bodies series. Cibachrome photograph, 120 × 120cm. Courtesy of the artist and Roslyn Oxley9 Gallery, Sydney.

still keep up, even though I was sick. We still don't have sex but don't tell anyone about it.

For Rick, too, sex was a problem:

> That is the one area at the moment that I'm having problems with. I have spoke to the doctor about it, and he says there is nothing there to say that anything should change, but he is looking at that at the moment. Because I'm, sort of, not ... haven't got the drive I had before, and I'm having a few problems with that. My wife says, "'Look, don't worry about it," all this sort of thing. But I honestly don't know, I think probably deep down, it does matter. Because, you know, we have been very active, and we are still very, very, close.

The Future Rehearsed

The external body ruptures and dysfunctions contribute to and are a metonym of the emotional challenges with which people deal following trauma or acute illness. The wound, scars, stumps, gaps and absences are ever-present mnemonics of the body's history; an artificial limb or an external breast, a stoma, an internal prosthesis are all literally surface tensions that are further reminders of corporeal change. Interior changes, such as those associated with organ and tissue transplants, are more difficult to think of in material terms, and partly for this reason, the attribution of behavioral change to cellular memory has an attraction. The changes to the body that occur with transplants are not on but below the surface; in many cases, even the scars are out of sight. Yet those who have had transplants must incorporate into their conceptualization of their own body the tissue or an organ that had another history. Human flesh cannot be sloughed off as material alone, in contrast to the ceramic, titanium, acrylic and stainless steel spare parts now used routinely in restorative surgery. Individual psychology interacts with cultural constructions of the body and affects the ability to adjust to bodies that are changed through the introduction to other human parts. Some bodily components – blood plasma and whole blood, for instance – appear to have low symbolic value for most people, and few people are traumatized by their introduction and the notion of being sustained by another's body fluid. This is, conceivably, partly due to the loss of individuality through the pooling of blood and blood products, as well as to the fact that blood is given from a living donor and is replaceable. The comfortable attitude towards transfused blood contrasts sharply with the uneasiness towards body parts 'harvested' as a result of a death.

"The social body constrains the way the physical body is perceived," Mary Douglas noted five decades ago, "There can be no natural way of considering the body that does not involve at the same time a social dimension" (Douglas 1973:65). The recipients of living-related donor kidneys, and the donors, are mindful of the imbrication of the biological and social, and the potential tensions that can arise following donation among kin are mediated through establishing physical distance and through joking relationships. John left home, for example, to establish his physical independence after his transplant. Terry's son did likewise. Lisa's brother teases her that she has the "best" kidney. In contrast, as already described, people who have received cadaver transplants address the social body in relation to the fantasized identity of the donor, and on this basis, they ascribe a social life to the organ while reflecting on the donors' families and their putative kinship relationships with them.

Fiction both anticipates and extends this apparently amoral trade from that of a life for a death, to speculation on the life lost, to the idea of consubstantiation and multiple other existential puzzles. What if the skin color of transplantation were different, as in the Miracle of St. Cosmas and St. Damian, in which the gangrenous (white) leg of the Roman deacon Justinian is replaced with the healthy (black) leg of a (deceased) Moor (Figure 6.4)? The details – the ethnicity and twin relationship of the brother surgeons, the social positioning of the recipient, the politics of the surgery, the issue of race – all invite deconstruction.

More common are the stories, in print and film, which date from Orlac's conceit of a thieving hand and which find echoes in the lived experiences of people who take advantage of transplant procedures. The first single-hand graft, for instance, was performed on a New Zealander, Clint Hallam, who had lost his hand fourteen years earlier from a chain-saw accident while in prison. He became obsessed with gaining a replacement part. The details of his accident and his criminal history were not known at the time of surgery when he was constructed as a hero; when his history was made known, he was reconstructed as 'bad.' This in turn contrasted with his donor hand, which had, according to reports, come from a motorcyclist killed in an accident (and, dying before his time, was constructed as 'good'). The graft was amputated at the patient's request on February 2, 2001, for apparent medical reasons due to his failure to adhere to anti-rejection treatment and physiotherapeutic regimes (bad men are bad patients), to the reported relief of the surgeons and physicians who

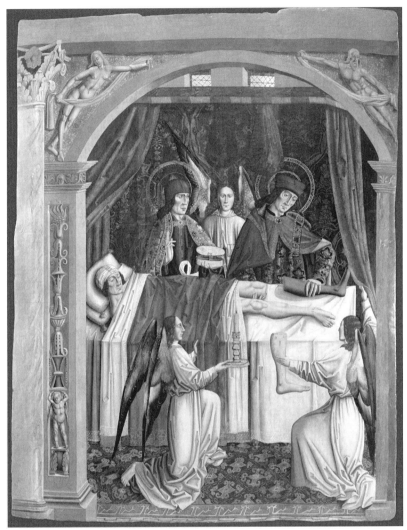

Figure 6.4 *A verger's dream: Saints Cosmas and Damian performing a miraculous cure by transplantation of a leg.* Oil painting attributed to the Master of Los Balbases, circa 1495. Courtesy of Wellcome Library, London.

had suffered an "exasperating two-and-a-half years" (Michelmore 2001). Around the same time, the Italian recipient of a transplant hand, tormented by its murderous history, requested that it be removed, too.

In presenting aspects of kidney transplantation, I have illustrated how individuals play a role in their surgical outcome, including by explicitly seeking or refusing to seek live-related donation. Here is the most explicit example of body politics: Can I give a part of my body to you? Can you accept a part of your body in mine? Anonymous cadaver donation circumvents this personal dilemma by replacing it with the unknown history of the donor and the organ. These dilemmas affect individuals' attitudes to their bodies, their ability to reintegrate their physical bodies, and to reintegrate their (remade) bodies/selves in society. This is another illusion: the replacement kidney must be routinely cared for by daily medication. While transplantation offers the recipient an illusion of normalcy, he or she is no less dependent on doctors, family and technology, particularly through medication to maintain immunosuppression, than are others whose semblance of normalcy is attained through visible and removable parts.

Note

1. This may reflect who initially chooses to proceed with a transplant. Gordon (2001, 2001) maintains that people who are especially uneasy about having someone else's organ are unlikely to accept transplantation as a treatment path.

7

Conclusion: Necessity's Children

Life and biology have their share of risks, as does life in society.
(Stiker 1999:12)

The public health revolution in the industrializing countries of Europe, dating from the early to mid nineteenth century, had a major and continuing impact on the incidence and distribution of disease. Breakthroughs in science at this same time, and the subsequent cascade in medical and technical innovations, also contributed to changes in epidemiology, demography and the social impact of disease. Conditions that were once life threatening increasingly became rare or minor events. Where wealth and technology coincided, death rates dropped dramatically. Over a century of incremental developments in biological knowledge and biotechnology mean that today the experience of illness and notions of being 'in good health' and 'fit' have changed substantially. Aches and pains, tiredness, shortness of breath, variations in eating and sleeping, declines in activities, energy and mood, once all regarded as 'normal' signs of aging, are now symptoms of pathology. Physicians and surgeons, among others, have gained increasing confidence in managing these signs and in marketing their skills and products. In industrialized societies especially, lives are created, sustained and extended by medical interventions that conquer individual vulnerabilities and the serendipity of biology. Pathologies and simple difference can be treated, re-aligned to be 'normal.' Transplantation, as one example, is an increasingly common way of intervening in a potentially fatal disease of essential organs when pharmacological or other therapeutic means are no longer productive. Worldwide, people have increasing access to the diagnostic tools and requisite surgical and chemical techniques to correct or halt pathological change and alleviate physical suffering.

In the face of illness, people search for a diagnosis; to name a condition is to begin to control it. The second step is to search for a cure, taking advantage of the proliferation of health services available from complementary and alternative modalities and cosmopolitan medicine. In a number of societies, including Australia, many services and technical interventions, including a wide range of drugs, are subsidized by the state, reducing the economic impact of various chronic conditions. Innovations, too, have stripped certain diseases of their social and potentially marginalizing impact. Insulin replaces the work of a non-functioning pancreas; lithium calms the embodied disruptions of a troubled mind; a pacemaker controls irregularities of the heart. External machinery and internal mechanics both support the human body: the dialyzing machine replaces the kidney; a cochlear implant in the inner ear processes and transmits sounds for people who are profoundly deaf; advanced methods for fertility control (injections and implants) and conception increasingly govern reproduction (Franklin and Roberts 2006; Franklin 2007). Biomedical interventions that initiate, maintain and enhance life and delay death are ubiquitous. Improvements in anesthesia, laser technology and key-hole surgery support economic imperatives to reduce inpatient hospital stays, increase day surgery rates and speed recovery. The near seamlessness of surgery and other, routine life events was unimaginable even a decade ago.

From the mid to late 1980s, a growing number of people requiring support and/or palliative care have been able to stay at home or in community facilities because of the development of equipment for home use, with or without the assistance of family, friends and community nurses. Home dialysis, ventilators and oxygenators, parenteral feeding pumps, medication infusion pumps, aspirators, humidifiers and nebulizers all support life in a home environment, converting the home to clinic while conversely (and perversely), hospitals are remodeled to seem homely. Many people would not survive without such equipment; their quality of life is improved when they are able to manage at home. Chapman and colleagues (1991) illustrated this nearly two decades ago with the example of a woman with terminal ovarian cancer and an inoperable bowel obstruction, for whom malnutrition and pain were both treated at home with parenteral nutrition administered through a central venous catheter, with the intestinal obstruction resolved with a endogastric tube draining into a leg bag. With night use of the equipment only, she stayed at home and remained active (it was claimed) until her death nine months later. People who are severely physically disabled and require ventilator-assistance and personal care similarly are able to live outside of institutions with noninvasive ventilation or with a tracheotomy, provided the caregiver can perform suction. Much of this home-care equipment requires reliable electricity. In some settings, electricity companies offer customers discounts while they use life-sustaining equipment, maintain registers of consumers using such equipment to ensure priority restoration of power supply in the event of power failure, and provide advice for a backup power source.[1] This does not happen in resource-poor countries, highlighting the inequities between rich and poor within and between countries.

The use of lung machines (Figure 7.1) and insertion of pacemakers are early cyborg innovations, but the extreme example remains the person declared brain dead and on life support; the ethics, politics and economics of continued support of a body with no possibility of regaining consciousness has continually challenged anthropologists, ethicists and theologians (Taylor 1997; Lock 2001). The debate about brain death has focused the purpose of life maintenance, brought to public international notice with the U.S. Supreme Court case regarding continued life support for Terri Schiavo (Gostin 2005; Perry, Churchill, Kirshner 2005). The most usual example, other than short-term maintenance for organ and tissue removal, is a pregnant woman, declared brain dead following an accident, fatal infection or aneurysm but maintained on life-support to extend gestational life to maximize fetal outcome. Although the first case was in 1979, the number of cases worldwide has been limited, and each year, there are reports of life support which increasingly extend in duration for women who either have irreversible loss of total brain function or are in a persistent vegetative state, i.e. with preserved brain stem function but no cerebral function. The goal is to enable the fetus to develop until around thirty weeks' gestation to optimize survival after Caesarian delivery. The ethics debate relates both to the construction of a woman's body as an incubator, and, to a lesser degree, to the (as yet unknown) short and longer term physical and psychological outcomes for the infant. But there is a wide range of positions on theological, economic and social grounds, between and within religious and other communities. Strange bedfellows, the most radical scientists and faith-based conservatives have advocated for this kind of life support, with pro-life groups insisting, in pamphlets, in protests outside fertility control clinics, and on the internet, on the inviolability of the life of a fetus. In contrast, feminist scholars have seen it as stripping a woman of agency (Nelson 1994) and utilitarian ethicists (Singer 1994) have argued that quality should take precedence over sanctity of life.

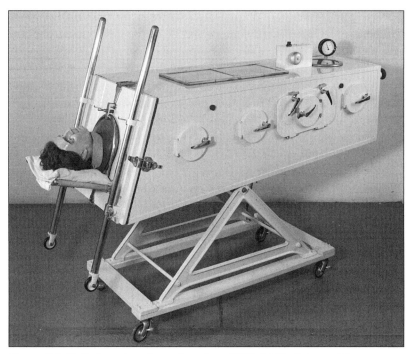

Figure 7.1 Both-type iron lung, London; 1950–1955; Science Museum, London. Courtesy of Wellcome Library, London.

The definition of death in countries such as the U.S. and Australia relates to brain, but elsewhere to heart and lung function (Lock 2004). Again, the nature of neurological activity raises ontological and moral concerns about consciousness and the quality of life. Jean-Dominique Bauby (1997), in his memoirs dictated with the flickers of an eyelid, attunes readers to the agility of a mind locked in a body that has lost all other independent functions. After a massive stroke in March 1997, Bauby lived for fifteen months with 'locked-in syndrome,' in which, as is characteristic, linguistic capability, intellectual and emotional functions remained intact but almost all motor abilities of self expression were lost. Like others with locked-in syndrome, Bauby used eye-lid movement to communicate with and dictate to his amanuensis to write of his experience of imposed silence and immobility. An activist for his condition, Bauby founded the Association du Locked-In Syndrome in France shortly before his death.[2]

Building on these observations and the preceding chapters, below I return to and extend my discussion of questions around transplantation, and consider representations of change in human form and material culture. In this concluding chapter, I consider how the technical and cultural limits to human corporeality have been questioned, and I trouble the ways in which the conditions and values of contemporary life have shaped the management of individual bodies and the economies of social bodies and structures. We engage every day in body economies, as banal as the purchase of body products that offer superficial youth, and as fraught as the promise through surgery of an ordinary, normal life.

Stock and Flow

In the previous chapter, I summarized the development of transplant surgery as a prelude to discussing the experiences of men and women who had had kidney transplants or had donated a kidney. By the late 1960s, as noted, kidney transplant surgery had become relatively routine in most industrialized countries, and medical and surgical teams had developed successful procedures to enhance short and long term outcomes. Repeat transplants could now be undertaken if the first transplanted organ was rejected, and various radical 'cluster transplants' had been undertaken, such as stomach, small intestine, colon, pancreas and liver for children with short-gut syndrome or adults with hepatic, pancreatic or duodenal cancer. Simmons (1971) suggests that by the 1970s, technology had already outstripped social resources for the optimal use of organ transplantations. This was an argument taken up by Renée Fox and Judith Swazey (1992:xv), who reflected on the legitimacy of "spare part surgery," caricaturing surgeons as vulture-like and "ghoulish" in their approach to potential donors and the appropriate timing to "harvest" organs for cadaveric transplants: "It is the 'spare parts' pragmatism," they wrote, "the vision of the 'replaceable body' and limitless medical progress, and the escalating ardor about the life-saving goodness of repairing and remaking people in this fashion that we have found especially disturbing." The book was envisioned and presented as a swansong (although, as it transpired, this was not their final word).

Technically although not ethically, the importance of the timing of 'harvesting' organs and tissue, implicated in debates related to brain death, was in part resolved as cryonic techniques improved. The Organ Donors Association in Australia, a non-government non-profit organization concerned with educating Australians about donation to improve the donation rate, includes on its home page a table advising the approximate preservation times (that is, the 'shelf life') of body products: heart, and heart/lungs, four to six hours; pancreas, up to 20 hours; liver 12–24 hours, kidney 18–72 hours; corneas, up to ten days; bone marrow, varies; skin, bone and heart valves up to five years (Straw 2003). Given lengthy waiting lists for transplantations, however, few organs or tissues actually sit on the shelf. The waiting time for a kidney is estimated to be 3.8 years; 1.2 years for lungs. Yet, in Australia in 2010, only around 300 people donated organs – kidney, heart, lung, liver, pancreas and pancreas islets – providing approximately 20 percent of the number of organs needed for those on transplant lists. In the U.S., in contrast, where there is extraordinarily high spending on medical procedures, technology and pharmaceuticals for organ failure and tissue loss, an estimated 73,000 people are on waiting lists at any given time, and 12,000 kidney transplants take place annually. Fewer than 10 percent of people on waiting lists will die before a suitable organ is found.

Everywhere demand exceeds supply for body parts. In the language of the professional and government bodies monitoring tissue and organ donations and use, *stock and flow* is low. Kidneys are only an instance; worldwide, the supply and use of human body parts for transplantation surgery is inadequate for all solid organs (kidney, liver, heart, lung, heart/lung, pancreas, and intestine), tissue (bone, skin, cornea, and heart valves), and cells (bone marrow, cord blood, islet cell, fetal cells, stem cells, and altered cancer cells). The chronic shortage of organs is strongly implicated in the rising incidence of organ thefts and markets, and debates about the right to sell organs. In 1984, payment (or compensation) to families for cadaveric organs was outlawed in the U.S., but the sale of frozen human sperm, eggs and bone has continued to be permitted. The rate of donation is far too low for most people to avail of such surgery. Lock (2000, 2001) and Scheper-Hughes (2002, 2004) have taken similar critical stances in relation to attitudes towards people in vegetative states who are seen, by some, as simply acting as short-term biological support-systems for organs waiting to be matched; there is often persistent pressure on families of people on life-support to donate organs. The growing demand for body parts has fuelled the growth of 'spare-part' markets and, to meet supply, the theft of organs and tissue from cadavers, kidnappings, murder and profiteering in poor countries (Scheper-Hughes). The moral and ethical qualms about these developments have local meaning for those who are considering a transplant, or are related to others with diseased organs, when this is their only chance of survival when mechanical support ceases to be effective, or they wish to be independent of mechanical support.

In Australia, organ and tissue availability is covered by legislation which followed an enquiry of the Law Reform Commission (Australia 1977), with state and territory specific legislation introduced between 1978 and 1985. Financial compensation for organ donation is illegal. As Halstead and Wilson (1991) observed in an Australian Institute of Criminology Report on the shortage of organs and the legality of various procurement practices, "The success of human tissue transplantation has thrust what was previously considered the realm of science fiction into the 'here and now,' bringing with it the potential for macabre commercial exploitation of uninformed poor citizens of the Third World" (1). Halstead and Wilson were concerned specifically with gross breaches in human rights that were already occurring – in the late 1980s, early 1990s – as organ markets expanded in centers such as Mumbai, Hong Kong, Cairo and Manila. Here people have donated organs for cash, their reported willingness an elision over their acute poverty, but the evidence of organs stolen from people receiving 'exploratory surgery' is compelling. Women's organs are sold to meet dowry payments in India, corpses are dismembered without family permission, and as a business side-line, there is a thriving black market in immunosuppressive drugs in poor countries.[3] The Transplantation of Human Organs Act (No.42) was passed in India in July 1994 to curb living donor organ sales and related commercial dealings and to regulate the removal, storage and transplantation of organs.[4] But the traffic in organs is lucrative and global. As documented in scholarly publications and reported in national and local newspapers (Joralemon 1995; Scheper-Hughes 2001, 2002a, 2002b, 2004), there has been continued evidence of kidnapping, murder, the harvesting of organs from executed prisoners and hospital deaths, and the illicit sales of organs in various countries where there are the tertiary facilities to absorb a flow of organs of questionable provenance.[5] Not all reports are verified – the alleged sale of a kidney in Zurich through an internet auction house was probably a hoax – but even so, such stories add to concern regarding the ethics of transplant surgery (Anonymous 2000: F4).

Despite accounts of the illegal trade in organs, most transplantation occurs within the boundaries of the law, although primarily for the rich and mobile: from Japan and Papua New Guinea to Australia, Yemen to Egypt, Indonesia to Malaysia. Organs travel, too: donor organs are imported from New Zealand to meet the shortfall in Australia. This is necessarily a stop-gap measure, however, propelling continuing research and development in artificial parts and in xenotransplantation. While mechanical parts may contradict conventional esthetics of the body, at least they usually have a known provenance (excepting prosthetics sales on eBay). Like surgical and other medical developments, there is a long social and medical history of the development of mechanical parts and artificial bodies (Wood 2002), dating from the 1740s when Claude Nicolas Le Cat, France, head surgeon at a hospital in Rouen, built an artificial man to illustrate the anatomical structure of humans and the circulation of blood through the body. Research from the early twentieth century focused on human-to-human transfers and transplants, but experimental work to develop mechanical parts in human bodies gained momentum after World War Two, reflecting both incremental developments in science and technology and the demand created by wartime survivors.

Scientific research and the popular imagination have centered on the heart primarily because of demand: donated hearts are rarer than kidneys, for obvious numeric reasons and because live donation is not possible. In the U.S., around 105,000 cardiac patients require a heart transplant at a given time; only about 3,000 become available each year. The disparity of stock and flow is similar worldwide. The American Society for Artificial Internal Organs was established in 1954, and Akatsu (1971) claims that at its 1958 meeting, the first discussions were held on the possibility of experimental research to develop an artificial heart. The U.S. Artificial Heart Program Office of the National Institutes of Health was established in 1964. Within ten years, researchers had resolved a series of problems associated with difficulties in blood handling, mechanics and techniques of implantation. From the mid 1970s, as Fox and Swazey (1992:103–107) describe, Robert Jarvik and colleagues used animals (sheep and calves) to test the viability of the artificial heart. The model animals were duly anthropomorphized: "Alfred Lord Tennyson" set a 268 day record as a calf recipient of an artificial heart; Ted E. Baer (read it aloud) was the world record holder sheep artificial heart recipient, and lived nearly 200 days; calf Charles lived for 72 days with a Jarvik device before he received his twin Diana's heart in a transplant operation. Rather than being sacrificed to enable researchers to study the effects of the implant/transplant, Charles continued to live for three more years as a stud bull for a commercial dairy farm. When he died his organs were returned to the laboratory for analysis. Man (and it was) became the 'animal of necessity' as the next step in these developments, leading to a series of artificial heart surgeries.

A more recent development, presented as a temporary bridge for people waiting for a human donor for transplant, was the self-contained mechanical heart, the AbioCor. The first such heart, a small (one kilogram) polyurethane and titanium heart, was inserted at the Jewish Hospital, Louisville, Kentucky, in early July 2001 (Romei 2001). It had two ventricles, connected to the left and right atria of the patient, the aorta and the pulmonary artery, which carried oxygenated blood to the body and deoxygenated blood to the lungs on an alternating basis. The pump was maintained by lithium-ion cell batteries in a pack situated in the abdomen; these were continually recharged by an external battery pack, worn on a belt around the waist and transmitting energy via radio waves. In the abdomen, too, was an electronic microprocessor, the 'brain' of the heart, regulating pumping to meet the body's needs, adapting blood flow to increases and decreases in activity. The mechanical heart looked, worked and 'thought' like a real heart in a real body.

It is a quick leap in the imagination to artificial parts that 'think' more extensively and to artificial people who 'live.' A robotic walking frame was released onto the market in 1999 to assist in mobility for people who were frail and poor-sighted. Robots and virtual pets like Tamagotchi make the Barbie dolls and the crying, eating and peeing baby dolls of my daughter's childhood seem quaintly dated. Sony (2003) developed Aibo: the first two initials of the name stand for Artificial Intelligence, although the name also derives from the Japanese word *aibou*, pal or partner, because, Sony says, Aibo makes a great companion for people. The company reported the development rather breathlessly:

> Sony's Aibo, the robotic dog, can't do the laundry, but it can entertain company. Aibo learns new behavior by interacting with humans, and has software to simulate emotion and instinct: in a bad mood it won't do as it is told; in a good mood, it will show off its favorite tricks, like playing soccer. Its motions can be programmed through a PC link.

Sony built 15,000 robots and received 135,000 orders in the first few months of its release, selling 3,000 Aibos in twenty minutes when the product first went on the market. NEC's rival robot was the R100, "designed to live with you ... as a useful and lovable partner." While it did not look like a human or a pet, it could walk and talk, and with two cameras and three microphones, could recognize up ten people and control appliances via infrared.[6] From replacement parts, then, to replacement pets and replacement assistants or – the terror of *Stepford Wives* – replacement partners for modern dwellers: R100 can surf the net, and send video clips and e-mail in response to voice commands.

Imaginary Lives

As transplants have become increasingly common, various books, and films routinely rerun on television channels and airlines, have addressed the ethics and politics of medical science. *The Resurrection of Zachary Wheeler* (1971), for instance, dealt with cloning humanoids (known as 'somas') for organs for transplant as part of a global medical scam. The film anticipated both the extensive international trafficking in organs and debates related to in vitro fertilization (IVF) conception for bone-marrow transplants and related procedures. In *Race against Time* (2000), in order to save the life of his son who is alleged to be terminally ill, Jim Gabriel agrees to a deal: the fictional corporation Lifecorps will provide the boy with treatment at no cost, provided Gabriel agrees to die within a year to enable the corporation to harvest his organs. This is one variation of a futures market. Picoult's book (2004) and Cassavetes's film (2009) *My Sister's Keeper* make the same points. In another recent film, *John Q* (2002), the contemporary dilemmas of differential access to medical technology according to class and race are explored, so exposing the limits of health insurance schemes and health management organizations. The insurance

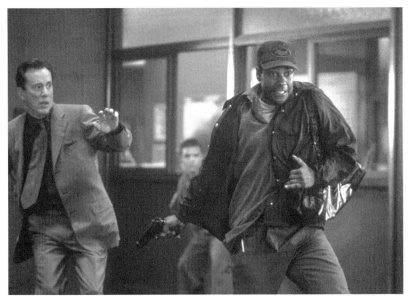

Figure 7.2 *John Q.*, U.S., director Nick Cassavetes; 2002.
Courtesy of Photofest.

company refuses to pay for a heart transplant for John Q's son; in despera-
tion, John Q holds the emergency room hostage. The film generated some
concern among health professionals, donor groups and other interest
groups worried about the impact of the film on people with terminal disease waiting for organs to become available, and on their families. Would
the film encourage copy-cat crime?

Film, literature and the visual arts critique and rehearse the possibilities for people with physical anomalies, organ failure and potentially
fatal disease, while they worry about the ethical and moral implications
of technology's uses and functions. So it is not coincidental that so many
popular films – at any given time, in any cinema – play with themes of
robots, transplants, transfers, clones, extraterrestrial beings, artificial
intelligence and the supernatural world. Lindsay Anderson's films *O
Lucky Man* and *Britannia Hospital,* discussed in chapter 2, reflect broad
cultural dis-ease with technology out of order and humans out of control; these are twentieth and early twenty-first century versions of Dr.
Frankenstein. Other films make light of such technical possibilities, and
instead bring to popular attention in simple language the theoretical
options of modern life. Consider *Junior* (1994), with its comedic representation of male pregnancy and the inevitable stereotypic development
of 'womanly' traits: "Feel my skin, isn't it soft?" And it allows a resolution, the marriage of the biological and birth parents and a subsequent
'normal' conception and pregnancy. Bioengineering and the impact of
anomaly (in this case, a man-born child) is thus reversed by the creation
of a conventional nuclear family. But, as Anne Balsamo (1996) argued
fifteen years ago, "Advances in reproductive technology already decouple
the act of procreation from the act of sexual intercourse," and the separation of gestation from the biological mother's womb has been explored
variously, including through surrogacy and post-menopause pregnancy.
Experiments of male pregnancy and lactation have not proceeded further
for social as much as technical reasons. However, the decoupling of biological and social parenting, in film (*The Kids are Alright*, 2010) and in the
lives of the famous, is increasingly commonplace.

Other films over the past half-century have played with ideas of sci-
ence-mediated metamorphoses, the extracorporeal creation of humans
and other beings, and cloning. Scientists tend to be portrayed as mad and
evil, and even when this is not so, the experimentation typically results in
disasters beyond human capacity. Some of the scenarios are Kafka-esque.
The Fly, made in 1958 and remade in 1986, deals with a scientist who

invents a genetic teleportation machine and begins to evolve as a human fly. In *Them!* (1954), atomic radiation interferes with the insect world, turning small ants into dangerous giant ants using the sewage systems of Los Angeles as an ant farm. In *Mimic* (1997), scientists seek to exterminate cockroaches with genetically-modified insects; these turn on humans as their next victims. *Mimic* is a rather apposite film in the twenty-first century, given vector and parasite mutation to insecticides and anti-helminths and the exploration of genetic modification of insects for this reason. But earlier films, too, were not so much prophetic as descriptive of the research achievements of the time, and their prophecies of doom were sometimes close to the mark.[7]

Reflections of the Future

Augmentative and alternative technologies have been developed and have established a market position as they have responded to social and economic changes, and to corresponding cultural shifts in the relationship of people to technological solutions. The ground work of transfer surgery and xenotransplantation was experimental and largely unproductive when artists and film-makers where shaping the science fiction of the limits of the body. Yet many of the innovations anticipated in fantasy have become common-place, pieces of equipment that are now no longer out of pocket, unnecessary, or invasive. Often the technical advances have resolved the embodied limits to function that have shaped exclusion and isolation. Advances in hearing aids, for instance, were propelled by the desire of people with incremental hearing loss as much as by scientists to disguise dependence on earlier forms of augmentative technology which underlined difference and marginality. But concurrently, a number of artists and industrial designers have appropriated and played with this technology to support resistance to both normalization and exclusion. Australian jeweler and designer Susan Cohn, for example, illustrates how good design enhances wearability and distracts – not detracts – from function: a hearing aid becomes jewelry to the point where it is unclear whether the aid is 'simply' jewelry or also an augmentative device. The same confusion between function and esthetic is ever present with my brace.

The DesignMensch exhibition – Designman: bodies, wrappings, surfaces in contemporary design – held at the Museum für Kunst unde Gewerbe in Hamburg in 2002 (Döring, Jockel, Joppien, Phillip, Strate 2001–2002) – built on this ambiguity between esthetics and function: its slogan was

Freud's (1930) *Der mensch – ein Prothesengott* (Man – A Prosthetic God), suggesting the ways in which prosthetics mimic and extend self-perception and provide the media for representation.

DesignMensch brings us full circle thematically. The exhibition explored the evolving symbiosis of body and technology. The body shapes and is shaped, enhanced and limited, by material culture; material and flesh interact in science and art, subject to shifts in esthetic taste, functional needs and bioengineering skill. Technology extends the body, and the body, in response to its own role in maximizing technical advantages, loses its spontaneity and other freedoms. The body is a hybrid. At its simplest, clothed, it is already encumbered and elaborated, protected and adorned. But at any given time, too, its biological structures are modified through connection to a robotic mechanism, a technology or a simple physical item (a wooden stick or a spoon, for example).

Many items at the exhibition were artifacts of everyday industrial life, examples of the contemporary history of material culture, body art and design esthetics, and irony and resistance. The exhibition included technologies of locomotion and communication, prosthetics and orthotics, ornamental and practical clothing, household items, and photographs of inscriptions on the body itself; it included implements that supplemented bodily skills, redressed deficiencies, extended capacity, and challenged constructs of assistive devices, the boundaries of design and the constitution of 'normal.' It included items for everyday use, often with the material side-products from space technology: lightweight, ventilated bicycle helmets from composite fiberglass with Kevlar and carbon fiber reinforcements to meet the demand for high speed travel and safety; motorbike helmets with Lexan visors; aluminum microscooters; lightweight and easily manipulated wheelchairs; exercise bikes. Items were prosaic, albeit exquisitely designed (a garlic press, a tea service), or whimsical or practical, items that had been worn once only or frequently: bracelets and necklaces, spectacles and hearing aids, ski wear and evening wear, garments structured to transform or fluid enough to follow the shape of the body, and other garments dyed and printed with computer images of the naked body so as to disappear altogether. There were masks and acrylic skeletons, and multiple other accoutrements of modern life – wrist cameras, micro CD players, video recorders, palm organizers, mobile phones, and so on. These display items were set against photographs of young contemporary urban dwellers, adorned with studs, rings, tattoos and brands, photomontages and photoshopped images, videos and displays of the human body on CD covers, calendars, catalogues, and annual reports.

The materials on display also reflected wider critical trends among artists in industrialized societies, and offered items that respond to contemporary needs – the tent is reshaped and extended, for instance, to meet the need for "mobility and flexibility" required by the "modern nomad"

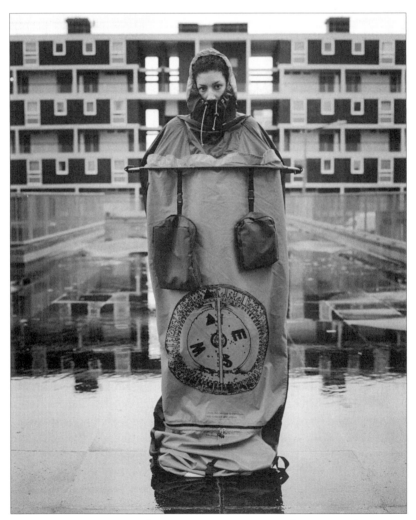

Figure 7.3 Lucy Orta, *Refuge Wear Intervention London East End 1998*. Original Lambda colour photograph, laminated, 150x120cm. Photograph by John Akehurst. © 2011 by Lucy+Jorge Orta. Courtesy of the artists.

(Bahlig and Bahlig 1996). The *Tentman* has much in common with the work of French artist Lucy Orta, who similarly emphasizes fluidity between clothing, transporting goods, and shelter. Her work, *Refuge Wear* (1992), was conceived initially for people in flight due to humanitarian crises or natural disasters; later works, including exhibitions in 2009 and 2010, have evolved to include street shelters for those who are homeless, and to explore in other ways the mechanisms for social transformation.[8]

Much art and practical items of contemporary design deal directly with disability and functional constraints. By their inclusion in this exhibition, and the growing attention to the narrow spaces between culture, esthetics and practicality, they challenge how we situate and conceptualize prosthetic and orthotic devices. The most routine pieces on display are ceramic ball-and-socket hip replacements, spectacles and, again, hearing aids. One on display, a silver behind-the-ear aid with a clear acrylic lead to the front of the ear and the canal, looked like a conventional hearing aid, simply much more elegant than the usual pink-plastic. The second was a tiny manikin sitting on the cartilaginous edge of the ear lobe, her back to an aid within the ear, her feet tucked into the fleshy lobe: the aid was a product from an industrial designer working in Germany to improve the technology, fitting methods, cost and service of hearing aids (Hörgeräte 2000).

The exhibition included also orthopedic supports from Rokitta, a Germany-based company that produces everything from lip balm, support hose and sportswear to grass cutters and earth moving equipment, children's playgrounds and cockpits. Tim Brauns's artificial leg with integrated skate (*Rollthese*) suggests the technical possibilities of prosthetic limbs that, in their use, break the nexus of body loss and inability. Consistent with the theorizing behind the larger project "Prosthetics grow wings" (Brauns 1996), in this example, the artificial limb extended the body, allowing the wearer to step away from the esthetics and the limitations of the normal body, and opt instead for an alternative form, appearance and function that is, potentially, physically and psychologically liberating. The display also included an Otto Bock C-Leg (the computer leg), initially developed in 1997, which uses a microprocessor to monitor 'swing' and 'stance' movement in real time to enable the prosthetic leg to adapt to different walking speeds and provide knee stability – allowing it, in fact, to mimic the natural gait of a sound leg. This is a leg that thinks. Thus, depending on the clothing that disguises or discloses, the possibility of stigma, exclusion and discrimination is perverted: its wearer is indistinguishable from other, 'normal,' folks.

Stelarc was represented in the DesignMensch exhibition, not surprisingly, given its futuristic perspective and his own studio in Hamburg. His pieces on display and his videos dramatized the paradoxes of extending the human body. The motion prostheses, the pneumatic operations involved in the performance of the Exoskeleton, the lighting both for the performance and film, the software development, filming and editing, the project coordination, and the compilation of this material for display, all highlight the collaborative nature of his art. The videos in particular demonstrate the interdependence of the performer and machines – the machines do not have an artificial intelligence independent of the artist (see also http:// web.stelarc.org). They are cumbersome and limited. Stelarc's third hand has only three degrees of freedom – pinch release, grasp release and wrist rotation – and is an encumbrance, a mass that impedes the sleek efficiencies and economies of the ordinary fleshy human body.

Stelarc had illustrated the alternative: the body controlled by a machine. In his earlier Ping Body performances (1996), dating from Sydney gallery performances, he used three computers, three cameras, two video projectors, a vision switcher, a vision mixer, a specialized sound system and the Internet. Subsequently, through the interface of his body and multiple computers, he was able to stimulate the body externally through Internet activity, rather than internally via the nervous system, while concurrently, he was also able to activate the robotic Third Hand to trigger the upload of images to a website. The role of impersonal collective activity on embodied movement led Stelarc to reflect that "the Internet (had become) not merely a mode of information transmission, but also a transducer, effecting physical action" (Stelarc 1996). In later work, Stelarc (2002) has pushed the notion of the hybridity of the body and machine, with the two working in temporary mutuality to produce effective locomotion. But the Exoskeleton is a corrective to cyborg fantasies: the six-legged pneumatically powered robot can move only with Stelarc and is limited by his physical capacity. Stelarc in turn is limited by the mechanical extensions. Attached to the machine, he is clumsy, robotic in ways reminiscent of old film footage, supra- rather than superhuman. Stelarc sees the interactions of the body with technology as a reflection of the relationship of body and machine in everyday relationships, such as playing a piano, using a keyboard or driving a car, where the body actively manipulates or navigates with these technologies. But the most obvious correlate is the use of muscles to 'work' prosthetics – the shoulder and back muscles enable the flexion of a hand in a prosthetic arm, for instance.

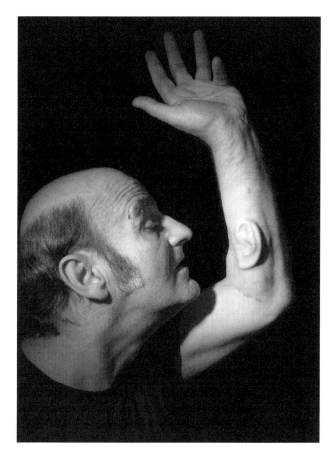

Figure 7.4
Stelarc, *Ear on
Arm*. London,
Los Angeles,
Melbourne;
2006.
Photograph by
Nina Sellars.
Courtesy of
Stelarc.

Stelarc's most recent projects retain this concern with excess rather than lack, resulting in collaboration on the extra ear. He began with an additional digital ear, demonstrated on his website, and he has since worked with scientists at Curtin University (Australia) using tissue engineering techniques to create the architecture of a third ear, implanted into his inner left arm for integration. This is a work in progress; the insertion of a microphone to convert the flesh into a 'hearing' ear the next step. His more recent work, meanwhile, has been to create quarter-scale ears from stem cells, able to exist without attachment as an example of 'partial life' and as a commentary on the manipulability of living systems and life itself.

Is the Body Obsolete?

> In the spheres of biological reproduction, genetic engineering and
> medical interventions of many sorts, the body is becoming a
> phenomenon of choices and options. These do not affect the individual
> alone: there are close connections between personal aspects of bodily
> development and global factors. Reproductive technology and genetic
> engineering … are parts of more general processes of the transmu-
> tation of nature into a field of human action. (Giddens 1991:8)

The commercial spin-offs are attractive to those backing biomedical
research and engineering advances, provoking trenchant criticism of
trends that feed into anxieties about ableism and the continued intolerance
and discomfort of those whose bodies from birth or over time vary from
the norm. In this section, I reflect on the commercialization of the body
beautiful before returning to the everyday activities and physical needs
that inspired these inventions. Early in this book, I noted how advances
in plastic surgery, supported by social values that favor youthfulness, have
become increasingly available as a dimension of cosmetic consumerism.
The internalization of an image of the self as distorted, ugly or fat has been
addressed extensively in the literature in relation to anorexia nervosa, in
other accounts of cosmetic surgery, and certainly, most poignantly, in
autobiographical accounts of reconstructive surgery, as described by Lucy
Grealy (1994), for instance.

The trend of what we might characterize as medical airbrushing
draws attention to the need to understand how cultural constructions of
the body propel people towards major surgery to effect bodily change,
and what this reveals about contemporary notions of health and wellbeing. Improvements in diagnosis and treatment of illness have shifted our
expectations of being healthy. We have come to expect, with industry's
encouragement, the absence of the superficial signs of aging, and to regard
as problematic and remedial body changes that are discordant with societal ideals of beauty, youth, slimness and fitness. In Australia and in the
United States in recent years, older women and men have been the particular targets of the marketing of cosmetic surgery and procedures, with
advertising aimed at an aging population that is self-conscious of 'middle
age spread,' wrinkles, sunspots and other blemishes. Any magazine or
newspaper will illustrate this. My suburban throw-away newspapers each
week advertise services that (in their words) promise to remove sagging

flesh and excess fat under the chin and across the stomach, and fill crevices and wrinkles – crow's feet and laugh lines – with this fat, remove 'love-handles' and stretched skin, get rid of unwanted hair, slim down thighs, strip out varicose veins, remove freckles and age spots from hands and face, and so on. These minor miracles draw on an extraordinary repertoire: 'laser' surgery, 'micro-current technology,' electrolysis, dermabrasion, and other non-surgical treatments that include aromatherapy, massage and ionized gels to tighten the buttocks, face, arms, stomach, neck, and legs. Teeth may be improved with esthetic porcelain, jaws broken and rejoined, chins realigned. But the promise is more than remedial – "*Become* the figure you always desired." The corporeal body and the self are one and the same.

Julie Rrap's art sharply criticizes this trend towards sculpturing the body to fit the cultural mold. Sometimes her work is fanciful, but it is often disturbing and sometimes repelling. Rrap uses photographic images and Photoshop techniques to interrogate popular culture, manipulating images to tease out the links between the real and imaginary. The piece that won the Hermanns Art Award 2002 is a case in point. *Overstepping* (Figure 7.5) is a digital print of human feet, morphed to have fleshly high heels. The work references genetic engineering as well as questions of fashion and fetishism, body modification and women's oppression (Alexander 2002). The artificial stance in a stiletto, in the absence of the 'natural' high heel, is precisely why hammer toe and mullet toe surgery are now such common procedures.

A number of other artists have used digital photography to fuse images and create interspecies, as illustrated in the *Artlink* special issue, *The Improved Body: Animals and Humans* (Britton 2002). Similar work of wit and irony circulates without identification or attribution by email or lives a limited life on the net, and so cannot be reproduced. These include various edited photographic images of consubstantial human, animal, plant and other natural forms. One especially clever web site, entitled *The Progressive Amputee*, is no longer maintained: a slide show of a man – an icon of bodybuilding – and a disappearing body. He begins with a prosthetic foot; through the series of images, his body parts are replaced, one by one, with prosthetic parts: his lower limbs, then upper limbs, then trunk. The final 'amputee' is a head on plastic. UK artist Alexa Wright pushes her work further, placing her own head onto the photographs of bodies of people with a variety of physical conditions (scoliosis, achondroplasia, congenital amputation) in order to challenge constructions of normality.

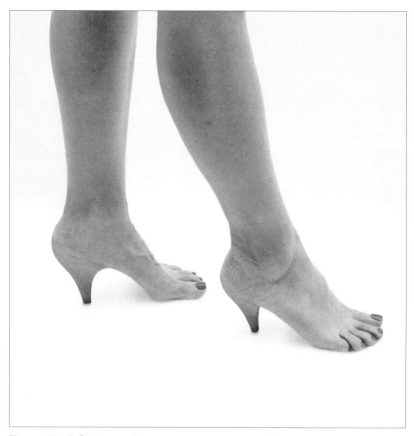

Figure 7.5 Julie Rrap. *Overstepping*; 2001. Digital print, 120 × 120cm.
Courtesy the artist and Roslyn Oxley9 Gallery, Sydney.

Excess presents a similar problem: consider heavy facial hair or baldness on women, or an extra digit.

By the early twenty-first century, film, art and design were increasingly teasing the potential of hybridity, as the work of artists such as Patricia Piccinini illustrates. This interest in playing with corporeality and genesis is old, of course, represented persistently in tales of the ancients and in medieval gargoyles, in depictions of xenogenesis, mutation and surrealism from Bosch to Dali, Kahlo and Magritte, as well as in children's books, in cartoon fantasy and science fiction. The theme of metamorphosis is recurrent. *Star Trek* and others of this genre, like the speculations on man-made

men in Lindsay Anderson's films, sustain much older themes of transformation and transfiguration in art and science.

Piccinini's works reference the scientific experiments involving xenotransplantation, but also the endless possibilities of imaginary species and
cross-species reproduction, and so capture the ethical dilemmas and anxieties of uncontrolled experimentation, modern-day re-workings of mad
science experiments and bodily fragments. *Beyond our Kin*, her most recent
exhibition of work, was shown in Sydney in late 2010, and in achieving its
disquiet, she uses silicone, human hair, animal pelt, fiber glass, steel – mix-
ing materials to illustrate the contradictions and tensions between human
reproduction, bodily structure, and technology. One example from the
exhibition is *The Comforter* (2010) – a sculpture of a prepubescent girl, covered in hair, cradling an indeterminate being, human infant-like in skin and
unrecognizable in the arrangement of limbs and organs. This work, Piccinini claims, is "one of the most optimistic works" in this exhibition of the
ethics of intervention in the "structure of life" (2010). Certainly it is a gently
empathetic work, against other less forgiving works that depict grotesque
infant-like bodies of a toxic world or of experimentation gone wrong: *Lit-
ter* (2010), three infants, humanoid but not human, huddled together like
newborn pups; and *Newborn* (2010), a humanoid hybrid with misshapen
limbs and a proboscis of unclear origin, nestling on a possum pelt. Several of these new works echo her earlier disturbing work, especially *We are
Family,* exhibited in the Venice Biennale in 2003. They also reference *The
Young Family* (2002), *Still Life with Hybrids* (2002) and *Leather Landscape*
(2003), portraits of imagined beings with denuded beagle ears and simian
tails, meerkat postures, suckling their young like piglets. But they are pink-
fleshed with Caucasian human hair. This is an imagined world gone wrong.
Julie Rrap's work is ironic, often wry; Patricia Piccinini's, in contrast, is a
frightening augur of a future uncontrolled.

Concluding Remarks

This is the cultural context in which the men and women of this book
live. People whose lives are disrupted and whose bodies are immutably
changed must adjust to a new manner of embodiment that is discrepant
with cultural norms, and readjust their sense of self in terms of their body
and its match with how others see and interact with them. They often live
marginalized and excluded at various levels, including by self-exclusion,
as both people with stomas and women with mastectomies demonstrate

so powerfully in describing their internalized notions and anxieties of the abject body. Changes in corporeality and the experience of embodiment disrupt and force reconstructions of personhood, the social self, social identity and relations with others.

The sophistication and effectiveness of public health and clinical interventions in industrialized societies limit the disruptiveness of disease for individuals and their families. For those whose lives are profoundly disrupted by chronic illness or trauma, surgery may be a last resort or an essential measure to ensure continued life. In some cases, the measures are extreme. The use of transplants as an alternative to mechanical or chemical control vividly illustrates the perceived desirable outcomes of diagnosis and care of disease: that is, the promise that after surgery the person – with her new heart, kidney, or liver – will be 'as new,' with the expectation that surgery will prolong life, enhance its quality, free the individual from biomechanical dependency, and reduce the need for surveillance and management. These are developments that were characterized by Renée Fox and Judith Swazey (1992:6) as auguring in a "new period of optimism." Such optimism informs the science behind new procedures and products, and shapes the narratives of renewal for people post-surgery. But adaptation to bodily change and the consequent reshaping of identity is hard work.

The normal is a cultural construct, and so the things that happen to bodies that are constitutive of abnormality vary. Stiker argued that "a society reveals itself by the way in which it treats certain significant phenomena" (1999:14). The 'problem' of disability is one. How such phenomena are treated, of course, depends on various other social cleavages and inequalities. Race, ethnicity and age are sharp lines of disadvantage. So is gender. As I have illustrated, bodies are gendered, and gender does not dissolve with disability or illness; rather, it provides one way of both receiving and doing disability. A striking outcome of the interviews with women and men was how, despite variations in physical condition, lived experience and response, and variations in embodiment post-surgery, gender made the difference. Gender for Sara was insinuated in her internalization of ideal body size, but also in her ideas of beauty that were disrupted irrevocably with stoma surgery and the scars across her abdomen. For others, the articulation of gender was clearest and least surprising when the surgical site was sexed, as with breast cancer, but the social construction of gender is so powerful that its template surfaced in all experiences.

As I have illustrated, women have attributed gendered meanings to various body parts. Drawing on a feminist framework, Ann – who had had both breast cancer and a hysterectomy – argued that giving birth was central to her sense of self, but also, that it was a generic, uniquely female act of embodiment. She saw her hysterectomy – the ripping out of her womb – as the price she paid for stepping outside of the boundaries of being female, causing conflict with her husband and children. Ann perhaps was overstating the analogy between embodied integrity and domestic harmony, but other women also explicitly linked their identity as women to their bodies, and so placed great symbolic weight on the loss of body parts. As illustrated, women spoke of being vulnerable without their breast(s), and violated, and also talked of feeling *a wholeness returned* with reconstructive surgery: "Without it," said one woman, "you don't feel a real lady, and of course you are not." Other women feel that their post-surgical bodies were "visually unpleasant for other people."

These gendered narratives and strategies do not rest with engendered embodied parts. Regardless of medical procedure, women continually picked up the narrative threads of the importance of the maintenance of femininity, and the use of prosthetic devices and tricks of the trade (of being female) to disguise the disruptions. Alison used an orthotic brace to walk, in order to appear and to *feel* less disabled than she felt when she was in a wheelchair; she wore clothing to disguise muscle wastage. Cathie wore a wig to disguise baldness and a prosthesis to disguise her mastectomy, and many of the woman – regardless of operation and resultant disability – spoke of dressing to look good, of wearing make-up, "putting on a face" and taking care of themselves in order to look as "normal as you can." There was resistance, too. Jane's was through private irony; she dressed in ways that drew attention to bodily parts that were problematic, highlighting for herself her ability to pass. A string bikini or a tight short skirt drags the eye of the other to the region of the body that is not what it seems – no anus, a colostomy, a urethra that has to be catheterized. Women's normality then can be a surface thing. The intent is to look as much as to be normal.

Gender performance for men focused on the things that they could do to be men, rather than on how they looked. I explored this particularly in the chapter on amputation and loss of body function, but the same themes emerged in interviews with men who had had stoma surgery and with men who had had transplants. Men must often deal with impotence as a consequence of their health condition or lifesaving medication. While this theme was constant, men also defined masculinity more broadly than women did femininity, and consistently emphasized action and achievement. Masculinity was embodied and internal; femininity was on the surface, exposed to the scrutiny of others. The man whose body had been broken needed to find a means of restitution, but this was almost always on a physical pathway. By involvement in everyday, masculine-associated pursuits, men identified and confirmed their survival. They refused to adapt their work routines and practices following surgery, because of a feeling that this would be 'giving in' to the disease. Normality was re-established by returning to a 'normal' routine, and men spoke of "*doing* as much as the others, *doing* more than my share." As one man, cited in chapter 3, explained: "I've got to go the extra step in most things" in order to re-establish normality.

The interpretation of normality according to gender is only one way in which we might think of surface tension as a metaphor for body catastrophe, degeneration, rupture, or simply change. In the individual accounts presented in this book, I have taken different instances of surface and substrata, exterior and interior, to focus on how changed corporeality affects individuals. The employment of surface as a heuristic device is clearest for people who have had an amputation, or who have other impediments affecting mobility and motility. As both Kath Duncan and Ju Gosling have recognized in their own work, it is not easy to hide a back brace or foreshortened limb without hiding yourself; their resolution of this conundrum was to resist dominant constructions of the normal that privilege particular appearances and types of bodies and treat personal worth, mental and physical capacities as isomorphic. The absence of body parts and visible dependence on a prosthesis or orthosis are surface evidence of people who breach social norms. External parts – the body and the appurtenances that might be needed to facilitate social participation – influence how individuals view themselves as social beings. In analyzing this, I have highlighted the problematic of the person and the body, the breaches of the body metaphorically reflecting how biology manipulates the social person. The wheelchair or the prosthetic limb, for instance, extends the body's boundary and imposes body loss into social settings and spaces, and so inserts the person as a social actor.

Contemporary industrialized societies such as Australia are not especially tolerant of bodies that deviate, that are smaller, fatter, differently proportioned, or that function or look different from others – as if physiological function, the capacity for pleasure, life chances and personal worth were all associated with size and appearance. In my second example of surface tension, I used men and women whose internal systems have failed to function or have become diseased, and who must necessarily manage the elimination of internal waste entirely manually, with the plumbing pipelines of their bodies brought from the inside to the surface. The stoma, indeed, is a procedure of inside to outside, the colon brought to the stomach as the flesh with which to create a new opening. The body is used to create its own replacement parts. The products of elimination are not unfamiliar, but excretion is a private and transitory thing, managed behind or beneath us – not at the front. This is only one anomaly. As I illustrate in chapter 4, men and women lose social adult status with loss of continence, and rehabilitation and adjustment following stoma surgery is both about managing the appliances and minimizing the discovery of their presence by others. The rituals of maintenance of the stoma inhibit the integration of the individual 'made well' with surgery. Stomas are ever-present and always in need of management.

Mastectomy is a particular form of amputation, and the surface tensions for women are significantly over-determined by gender. The below-surface tension is the cancer itself. But, as I illustrated in relation to women who had had prophylactic mastectomies following genetic diagnosis, the tension is in the molecular basis of the body itself. Women's accommodation to breast loss did not make up for the essential assaults on their personal identity and self-confidence that occurred as a result of the surgery and its surface memories: the scars, the concavity of chests, the puffiness of edema. Women were often shocked by the integral links between body and self that were disrupted with the loss of a breast. Am I so superficial, women asked, that being two-breasted matters so much to me?

My final example involved multiple tensions of surface and substance. People who survive after kidney failure, or as their kidneys weaken, must accept a mechanical means to take over the work that kidneys usually do autonomically. Hemodialysis takes the inside out; peritoneal dialysis takes the outside in. In enabling this mechanical management of the body – the washing of blood, a task almost unimaginable in everyday language, for *can liquid be washed?* – the surface of the body, too, must be changed. The creation of a fistula for hemodialysis or a stoma for peritoneal dialysis in turn creates a new sense of embodiment, forcing people to adjust to and care for the body in profoundly different new ways. A renal transplant carries the idea of a tension between the surface and interior body, and relation of body to self, even further. In contrast to the person who must 'wear' his or her wheelchair or prosthetic limb(s), the transplant recipient is even more dependent on external technology. Individual responses to transplantation surgery vary according to perceptions of justice and agency, in terms of how the event leading up to surgery is construed and the degree that the individual was able to influence the surgical outcome. This in turn affects their attitudes to their bodies, their responsibility for body maintenance and performance, the reintegration of their bodies, and the reintegration of their (remade) bodies/selves in society. With renal transplant, the replacement kidney must be checked routinely. Its viability depends also on the person adhering to immunosuppressant medication to prevent the body turning on itself. Free from mechanical dependency, the person is now, instead, dependent on the effective workings of a body part that brings with it its own history (of the body of another); and while the kidney itself is buried below the surface, the medication that ensures its harmonious residency is not hidden in the body system. Steroids mark the body with weight gain and hirsuteness, etching on the surface the body's frailties, after all.

I have teased out and contrasted manipulations of body surface and reconstructions of bodily boundaries, with responses to and management of undesired corporeal changes. In bringing together diverse examples of 'exceptional' rather than 'normal' bodies, I have searched for commonalities in the meanings of corporeality for people whose disabilities, anomalies and transformations have been beyond their control. I have searched, contrarily, for commonalities in the meanings of normality for those who have had no choice but to negotiate their corporeality. In *Modernity and Self-Identity*, Giddens (1991:7) explores the contemporary project of reflexivity of the self, in which he suggests a concern to construct and control the body that underpins what he characterizes as "the narcissistic cultivation of bodily appearance." The exercise of will by people with anorexia in denying appetite, and so controlling both bodily desire and morphology, provides a sharp illustration of how people seek to control the body. But the everyday engagements of technology and the body carry individuals outside of such self-reflexivity. There are no identity politics to complicate a reading of the use of the pacemaker, dialysis or a stoma bag, although people may find it difficult to come to terms with their need to rely on technologies in order to survive. A few of these technologies – breast prostheses and cochlear implants – are subject to cultural politics, particularly because they highlight normative ability and gender. Popular esthetics prescribe the normal body, and in so doing, prescribe prosthetics that are cosmetic as well as functional, 'normalizing' disabled people in an ableist world (Pernick 1997).

Ovid was one of many philosophers and writers fascinated by hybridity, mutation, deviance and transmogrification. So was Kafka. Fables and myths, manuscript borders and the parapet edges of cathedrals and theatres, circuses and science fiction films, are peopled with beings that resist the integrity of species and form. The vehicles for social criticism derive from such fancy, but so, too, does the experimental imagination. Its application leads to ways to resolve the perplexing, complex and mundane challenges of the body: to see more sharply, to maintain mobility without limbs, and to continue the bodily functions of digestion in the face of organ failure and tissue erosion. The solutions to bodily dysfunction provoke intense debate. Moral standpoints, cultural politics and social ideals inform discourse of the ethics and economics of medicine and the appropriateness and sustainability of specific procedures. The sharpest critics challenge the notions of normality that inform technologies of medicine, but those who take advantage of them do so precisely to live a life that is normal. In understanding the juxtapositions of ideology and material culture, we face recurrent questions, posed at the levels of both the individual and society. In this context, questions constellate around the social cost of illness and the values inherent in intervention. The debates typically seem theoretical. But people, and their mundane struggles with daily living, are real. The realities for people after injury or surgery are complicated and difficult, and involve singular journeys that often lack generosity in understanding from others. The resort to discourses of normality, and the efforts that are taken to align values and material circumstances, provide them with a securer pathway to move forward.

Notes

1. These kinds of services are offered as a selling feature to customers in competitive markets, e.g. in the United States; see web pages of electric companies such as the Salt River Project (Central Arizona) and Midwest Electric (Ohio).

2. The association provides community education, research and social support, and supports ergotherapy with various technical devices to facilitate communication and allow access to some autonomy for people with locked-in syndrome to live a "second life" (Association du Locked-in Syndrome 2003).

3. The authors (6) proposed various alternatives to meet demand other than presumed consent, including the introduction of a futures market in cadaver organs as "the most palatable form of organ commerce," whereby individuals could elect to donate body parts upon death, for financial consideration while alive and in good health, which they argued would allow the decision to donate to be made rationally. Payment could be made to a charity of choice, the authors suggested, thereby maintaining the fiction of altruism. To my knowledge, suggestions from the report were taken no further.

4. However, it is legal under the enactment to reimburse a donor the direct and indirect costs of supplying an organ, including loss of earnings, and there is provision for non-related living donations of organs.

5. For instance, in Thailand in late 1999, allegations were made of illegal trading in organs in Vachiraprakan Hospital, leading to the reopening of an investigation into the potential murder of the nurse who allegedly "knew too much" about the trade. Her death earlier in the year had previously been determined accidental (Anonymous 2000:A2).

6. For details of R100, see NEC's website http://www.incx.nec.co.jp/robot/R100/. A quick search of the web in 2010 indicates an extraordinary number of humanoid robots.

7. Consider, for instance, the rapid loss of toxicity of DDT against mosquitoes, and the rapid evolution of and resistance to the myxoma virus.

8. Modular Architecture, for example, allows four individuals to travel separately by day in waterproof, insulated, hooded body-suits made of aluminum-coated polyamide, with pockets for water storage, food and medicine; at night the garments convert into a single tent to accommodate all four, empty limbs of the tent now the means by which the dwelling is secured. The production of this work is itself often transformative. Her Melbourne residency in April 2002, entitled "Art as an Agent of Social Change," brought together other artists, students and local residents to construct fluid environments around the themes of belonging ("Heart") and connection ("Nexus") (Manderson, fieldnotes April 2002; for project notes, see http://studioorta.free.fr/life_nexus/projet.html, accessed 28 March 2003).

References

Abram, H. S. and D. C. Buchanan (1978). "Organ transplantation: psychological effects on donors and recipients." Medical Times 88: 23d–29d.

Abu-Duhou, J. (2002). Violence against women in Ramallah, Palestine. Key Centre for Women's Health in Society, Department of Public Health. Melbourne, Australia.

Acierno, R., H. S. Resnick, and D. Kilpatrick (1997). "Health impact of interpersonal violence: Prevalence rates, case identification, and risk factors for sexual assault, physical assault, and domestic violence in men and women." Behavioral Medicine 23(2): 53–64.

Ades, M. J. (1993). The Wounded Woman. Bali.

Ades, M. J. (1995). Loss. Bali.

Ades, M. J. (1997). The Cancer Series. Paddington, Mary Place Gallery.

Akatsu, T. (1971). Artificial heart: Partial support and total replacement. *In* Human Organ Support and Replacement: Transplantation and Artificial Prostheses. J. D. Hardy, ed. Pp. 384–414. Springfield, IL: Charles C.Thomas.

Alexander, G. (2002). "Sex in the cyborg: Julie Rrap's Overstepping." Artlink 22(1): 27–31.

Anderson, L. (1968). If, UK and U.S., Paramount: 111 minutes.

Anderson, L. (1973). O Lucky Man, UK and U.S.,Warner Brothers: 183 minutes.

Anderson, L. (1982). Britannia Hospital, UK, EMI: 116 minutes.

Anonymous (1998). Master Breasts. Mariogros, Italy: Aperture Foundation.

Anonymous (2000). "Suspicion over death of nurse." The Nation (Bangkok) (February 29).

Anonymous (2002). "Full face transplant no longer a fantasy." The Nation (Bangkok): 9A.

Ardener, S. (1987). A note on gender iconography: The vagina. *In* The Cultural Construction of Sexuality. P. Caplan, ed. Pp. 113–142. London and New York: Tavistock Publications.

Arnesen, T. and E. Nord (1999). "The value of DALY life: Problems with ethics and validity of disability adjusted life years." British Medical Journal 319(7222): 1423–1425.

Art.Rage.Us. (2001). "Artists and Writers." Retrieved April 8, 2003, from http://www.breastcancerfund.org/artrageus_artists.htm.

Ashby, H. (1978). Coming Home. U.S., United Artists: 126 minutes.

Association du Locked-in Syndrome (ALIS). (2003). Paris. http://www.alis-asso.fr/.

Australia, Department of Health and Aging (2006). "2006 National Competition for Organ and Tissue Donation." Retrieved May 6, 2007, from http://www.health.gov.au/internet/wcms/publishing.nsf/Content/health-organ-comp2006.htm.

Australia, Department of Health and Aging (2007). "2007 National Competition for Organ and Tissue Donation." Retrieved May 6, 2007, from http://www.health.gov.au/organ-donation-comp.

Australia, House of Representatives. Standing Committee on Health and Aging (2009). Weighing it up: Obesity in Australia. Canberra: The Parliament of the Commonwealth of Australia.

Australia, Law Reform Commission (1977). Human Tissue Transplants. Canberra: Law Reform Commission.

Australian Broadcasting Authority (1999). Investigation Report: SBS TV "My One Legged Dream Lover" Documentary Promotion April 9, 1999, and Program April 14, 1999, "Sex And Nudity In 'G' And 'PG'." File No: 1999/0324. Complaint No: 10894. Investigation No: 700. Sydney.

Australians Donate: The Peak National Body for Organ and Tissue Donation for Transplantation (2007). Retrieved May 6, 2007 from http://www.australiansdonate.org.au/11650+0+home.htm.

Avary, R. (1996). Mr. Stitch. U.S., Thriller Production Co(s), Studio Megaboom and Rysher Entertainment: 98 minutes.

Bahlig, M. and Z. Bahlig (1996). Zelt-Jacke Tentman. Exhibition notes. Hamburg, DesignMensch Exhibition, Museum für Kunst und Gewerbe.

Balsamo, A. (1996). Technologies of the Gendered Body. Durham, NC: Duke University Press.

Bandyopadhyay, M. and M. R. Khan (2003). Loss of face: Violence against women in South Asia. *In* Violence against Women in Asian Societies. L. Manderson and L. R. Bennett, eds. Pp. 61–75. London: RoutledgeCurzon.

Bauby, J. D. (1997). The Diving Bell and the Butterfly. New York: Alfred A.Knopf.

Beckett, S. (1973). Not I. London: Faber.

Benhabib, S. (1992). Situating the Self: Gender, Community and Postmodernism in Contemporary Ethics. New York: Routledge.

Berger, J. (1972). Ways of Seeing. Harmondsworth, UK: Penguin.

Besson, L. (1997). The Fifth Element, France, Gaumont Film Company: 126 minutes.

Blacking, J., ed. (1977). The Anthropology of the Body. ASA Monograph 15. London: Academic Press.

Bourdieu, P. (1977). Outline of a Theory of Practice. Cambridge and New York: Cambridge University Press.

Bowes, A., T. S. Gingras, B.A.Kaplowitt, and A.Perkins, eds. (2000). Unbearable Uncertainty: The Fear of Breast Cancer Recurrence. Northampton, MA: Pioneer Valley Breast Cancer Network.

Braidotti, R. (1994). Mothers, monsters, and machines. *In* Writing on the Body: Female Embodiment and Feminist Theory. K. Conby, N. Medinam and S. Stanbury, eds. Pp. 59–79. New York: Columbia University Press.

Brauns, T. (1996). Rollthese. Exhibition notes. Hamburg, DesignMensch Exhibition, Museum für Kunst und Gewerbe.

Breast Cancer Answers Art Gallery (1996–1999). The breast cancer experience in images and words. Berkeley, Breast Cancer Answers Project, C/NET Solutions.

Brent, L. (1997). A History of Transplantation Immunology. San Diego, CA: Academic Press.

Britton, S. (2002). "The improved body: Animals and humans." Special issue, Artlink, Australian Contemporary Art Quarterly 22(1): 6.

Butler, J. (1990). Gender Trouble: Feminism and the Subversion of Identity. New York and London: Routledge.

Cabron, L. (2006, April 9, 2007). "They're Dreaming of a Boobs Christmas." 10 Zen Monkeys Retrieved December 5, from http://www.10zenmonkeys.com/2006/12/05/boobs-christmas-contest/.

Canguilhem, G. (1991). The Normal and the Pathological. New York: Zone Books.

Casey, E. S. (1987). Remembering: A Phenomenological Study. Bloomington: Indiana University Press.

Chapman, C., J. Bosscher, S.Remmenga, R.Park, and D. Barnhill (1991). "A technique for managing terminally ill ovarian carcinoma patients." Gynecologic Oncology 41(1): 88–91.

Cibelli, J. B., S. L. Stice, P.J.Golueke, J.J.Kane, J.Jerry, C.Blackwell, F.A.P. de Leon, and J.M. Robl (1998). "Cloned transgenic calves produced from nonquiescent fetal fibroblasts." Science 280(5367): 1256–1258.

Cimino, M. (1978). The Deer Hunter. U.S., Univeral Pictures: 183 minutes.

Cipolla, C. M. (1992). Miasmas and Disease. Public Health and the Environment in the Pre-Industrial Age. New Haven, CT: Yale University Press.

Cohen, L. (2001). "The other kidney: Biopolitics beyond recognition." Body and Society 7(2–3): 9–31.

Connell, R. (1995). Masculinities. Sydney: Allen and Unwin.

Corbin, A. (1986 [1982]). The Foul and the Fragrant: Odor and the French Social Imagination. Cambridge, MA: Harvard University Press.

Crouch, M. and L. Manderson (1993). New Motherhood: Cultural and Personal Transitions in the 1980s. Chur, Switzerland: Harwood Academic Press.

Csordas, T. J. (1994). Introduction: The body as representation and being-in-the-world. *In* Embodiment and Experience: The Existential Ground of Culture and Self, T. J. Csordas, ed. Pp.1–26. Cambridge, UK: Cambridge University Press.

Dahm, F. and M. Weber (2002). "History of Organ Transplantation." Life Sciences Zurich. Retrieved January 17, 2011, from http://www. lifescienceszurich.ch/focus2/history-en.asp.

Davidson, M. (2008). Concerto for the Left Hand: Disability and the Defamiliar Body. Ann Arbor: University of Michigan Press.

Davis, K. (1995). Reshaping the Female Body. The Dilemma of Cosmetic Surgery. New York and London: Routledge.

Davis, L. (1995). Enforcing Normalcy: Disability, Deafness, and the Body. London: Verso Press.

Davis, L. (1997). Nude Venuses, Medusa's body, and phantom limbs: Disability and visuality. *In* The Body and Physical Difference: Discourses of Disability. D. T. Mitchell and S. L. Snyder, eds. Pp. 51–70. Ann Arbor: University of Michigan Press.

de Moulin, D. (1983). A Short History of Breast Cancer. Boston: Martinus Nijhoff.

Deane, K., M. Carman, and M. Fitch (2000). "The cancer journey: Bridging art therapy and museum education." Canadian Oncology Nursing Journal 10(4): 140–146.

Del Toro, G. D. (1997). Mimic, U.S., Miramax: 105 minutes.

Deschamps, J. Y., F. A. Roux, P.Sai, and E.Gouin (2005). "History of xenotransplantation." Xenotransplantation 12(2): 91–109.

Dessaix, R. (1996). Night Letters: A Journey through Switzerland and Italy. Sydney: Macmillan.

Dick, P. K. (1968). Do Androids Dream of Electric Sheep? New York: Ballantyne Books.

Donaldson, R. (1995). Species, U.S., Metro-Goldwyn-Mayer: 117 minutes.

Döring, J., N. Jockel, R.Joppien, C.G. Phillip, and U.Strate (2001–2002). DesignMensch. Hamburg, Museum für Kunst unde Gewerbe.

Douglas, G. D. (1954). Them!,U.S., Warner Brothers: 94 minutes.

Douglas, M. (1973). Natural Symbols: Explorations in Cosmology. London: Barrie and Jenkins.

Douglas, M. (1978 [1966]). Purity and Danger : An Analysis of Concepts of Pollution and Taboo. London: Routledge and Kegan Paul.

Dovev, L., ed. (1996). Beauty is a Promise of Happiness. Catalogue of a One Woman Exhibition by Ariela Shavid. Jerusalem: The Israel Museum.

Duncan, K. (1999). My One-Legged Dream Lover. P. Fowler-Smith and C. Olsen. Sydney, Australian Film Alliance Corporation Limited, Dreamlover Film Proprietry Limited: 52 minutes.

Duncan, K. and G. Goggin (2002). "Something in your belly: Fantasy, disability and desire in My One-Legged Dream Lover." Disability Studies Quarterly 22(4): 127–144.

Eco, U. (2000). Kant and the Platypus: Essays on Language and Cognition. London: Vintage Books.

Edison, T. (1908). The Thieving Hand, J. S. Blackton Dir., U.S., Vitagraph Studios: 5 minutes.

Eikenberry, J. (1998). Introduction. *In* Art.Rage.Us.: Art and Writing by Women with Breast Cancer. San Francisco: Chronicle Books for The Breast Cancer Fund, The American Cancer Society (San Francisco Bay Area), and The Susan G.Komen Breast Cancer Foundation (San Francisco Chapter).

Eiseman, B. and A. Velasquez (1971). Extracorporeal and auxiliary liver support. *In* Human Organ Support and Replacement: Transplantation and Artificial Prostheses. J. D. Hardy, ed. Pp. 100–110. Springfield, IL: Charles C. Thomas.

Feinberg, T. E. (2001). Altered Egos: How the Brain Creates the Self. New York: Oxford University Press.

Ferguson, S. J. and A. S. Kasper (2000). Living with breast cancer. *In* Breast Cancer: Society Shapes an Epidemic. A. S. Kasper and S. J. Ferguson, eds. Pp. 1–22. New York: St Martin's Press.

Fisher, S. (1990). The evolution of psychological concepts about the body. *In* Body Images: Development, Deviance, and Change. T. F. Cash and T. Pruzinsky, eds. Pp. 3–20. New York and London: Guilford Press.

Flor, H. (2002). "Phantom-limb pain: Characteristics, causes, and treatment." Lancet Neurology 1(3): 182–189.

Foucault, M. (1977). Discipline and Punish: The Birth of the Prison. London: Allen Lane.

Foucault, M. (1978). The History of Sexuality. New York: Pantheon.

Fowler-Smith, P. D. and C. D. Olsen (1999). My One-Legged Dream Lover. K. S. Duncan, screenwriter. Sydney, Australian Film Finance Corporation Ltd. and Dream Lover Films Pty Ltd.: 53 minutes.

Fox, R. C. and J. P. Swazey (1992). Spare Parts: Organ Replacement in American Society. New York and Oxford, UK: Oxford University Press.

Frank, A. (1995). The Wounded Storyteller: Body, Illness, and Ethics. Chicago: University of Chicago Press.

Frank, A. W. (1990). "Bringing the bodies back in: A decade review." Theory, Culture and Society 7(1): 131–162.

Frankl, V. E. (1963). Man's Search for Meaning. New York: Washington Square Press, Simon and Schuster.

Franklin, S. (2007). Embodied Progress: A Cultural Account of Assisted Conception. New York: Routledge.

Franklin, S. and C. Roberts (2006). Born and Made: An Ethnography of Preimplantation Genetic Diagnosis (In-formation). Princeton, NJ: Princeton University Press.

Frawley, M. (1997). "A prisoner to the couch": Harriet Martineau, invalidism, and self-representation. *In* The Body and Physical Difference. Discourses of Disability. D. T. Mitchell and S. L. Snyder, eds. Pp. 174–188. Ann Arbor: University of Michigan Press.

French, L. (1994). The political economy of injury and compassion: Amputees on the Thai-Cambodia border. *In* Embodiment and Experience: The Existential Ground of Culture and Self. T. J. Csordas, ed. Pp. 69–99. Cambridge, UK: Cambridge University Press.

Gallagher, P., D. Allen and M. MacLachlan (2001). "Phantom limb pain and residual limb pain following lower limb amputation: a descriptive analysis." Disability and Rehabilitation 23(12): 522–530.

Gandy, M. (1999). "The Paris sewers and the rationalization of urban space." Transactions of the Institute of British Geographers NS 24: 23–44.

Garland-Thomson, R., ed. (1996). Freakery : Cultural Spectacles of the Extraordinary Body. New York: New York University Press.

Garland-Thomson, R. (1997). Extraordinary Bodies: Figuring Physical Disability in American Culture and Literature. New York: Columbia University Press.

Garland-Thomson, R. (2009). Staring: How We Look. New York: Oxford University Press.

Gawler, G. (1994). Women of Silence: The Emotional Healing of Breast Cancer. Melbourne: Hill of Content.

Gibson, W. (1984). Neuromancer. London: Gollancz.

Giddens, A. (1991). Modernity and Self-Identity: Self and Society in the Late Modern Age. Stanford, CA: Stanford University Press.

Girard, B. (1972). The Mind Snatchers, U.S.,Cinerama: 94 minutes.

Goffman, E. (1959). The Presentation of Self in Everyday Life. New York: Doubleday Anchor Books.

Goffman, E. (1963). Stigma. Eaglewood Cliffs, NJ: Prentice-Hall.

Goldberg, R. (2002). "Of mad love, alien hands and the film under your skin." Kinoeye 2(4): 1–7.

Gordon, E. J. (2001). "Patient's decisions for treatment of end-stage renal disease and their implications for access to transplantation." Social Science and Medicine 53(8): 971–987.

Gordon, E. J. (2001). "'They don't have to suffer for me': Why dialysis patients refuse offers of living donor kidneys." Medical Anthropology Quarterly 15(2): 245–267.

Gosling, J. (1997–2005). London, Ju Gosling. Retrieved June 6, 2011, from http://www.ju90.co.uk.

Gostin, L. O. (2005). "Ethics, the constitution, and the dying process – The case of Theresa Marie Schiavo." JAMA (19): 2403–2407.

Grealy, L. (1994). Autobiography of a Face. New York: Houghton Mifflin.

Greenwald, L. (2007). Heroes with a Thousand Faces: True Stories of People with Facial Deformities and Their Quest for Acceptance. Cleveland, OH: Cleveland Clinic Guides.

Grosz, E. (1994). Volatile Bodies: Toward a Corporeal Feminism. Sydney: Allen & Unwin.

Halstead, B. and P. Wilson (1991). 'Body Crime': Human Organ Procurement and Alternatives to the International Black Market. Canberra: Australian Institute of Criminology.

Hammond, C. (2001). "The epidemiology of cataract." Optometry Today: 24–28.

Haraway, D. (1991). Simians, Cyborgs and Women: The Reinvention of Nature. New York: Routledge.

Hertz, R. (1960 [1909]). Death and the Right Hand. London: Cohen & West.

Hill, A. (1999). "Phantom limb pain: A review of the literature on attributes and potential mechanisms." Journal of Pain and Symptom Management 17(2): 125–142.

Holm, D. K. (2002). "Britannia Hospital." The DVD Journal, Retrieved June 25, 2004, from http://www.dvdjournal.com/quickreviews/b/britanniahospital/q/shtml.

Hörgeräte, K. (2000). Frau in Ohr und Claro. Burgwedel, Germany: Hörgeräte KIND GmbH & Co. KG.

Hudson, P. (2003). E-sthetics. Albuquerque, NM: Patrick Hudson.

Huxley, A. (1983 [1932]). Brave New World. Harlow, UK: Longman.

iRobotics, I. (2003, March 26, 2003). "Home Page." Industries served. Retrieved March 29, 2003, from http://www.irobotics.com/industries.php3.

Isaksen, L. W. (2002). "Toward a sociology of (gendered) disgust." Journal of Family Issues 23(7): 791–811.

Jackson, C. (2002). Living Doll: The Amazing Secrets of How the Cosmetic Surgeons Turned Me into the Girl of My Dreams. London: Metro Books.

Jackson, J. (1994). Chronic pain and the tension between the body as subject and object. *In* Embodiment and Experience: The Existential Ground of Culture and Self. T. J. Csordas, ed. Pp. 201–228. Cambridge, UK: Cambridge University Press.

Jacobs, B. (1999) "Keeping the superstitions that work." The Yale Herald Online: Opinion 27.

Jenkins, J. H. and M. Valiente (1994). Bodily transactions of the passions: El calor among Salvadoran women refugees. *In* Embodiment and Experience: The Existential Ground of Culture and Self. T. J. Csordas, ed. Pp. 163–182. Cambridge, UK: Cambridge University Press.

Johnson, S. (1999). A Better Woman. Sydney: Random House.

Joralemon, D. (1995). "Organ wars: The battle for body parts." Medical Anthropology Quarterly 9: 335–356.

Kapsalis, T. (1997). Public Privates : Performing Gynecology from Both Ends of the Speculum. Durham, NC: Duke University Press.

Kasper, A. S. and S. J. Ferguson, eds. (2000). Breast Cancer: Society Shapes an Epidemic. New York: St. Martin's Press.

King, S. E. (1997). Treading the Maze, An Artist's Journey Through Breast Cancer. San Francisco: Chronicle Books.

Krawczyk, G. (2004). Transplanting Memories. NZ, TV documentary: 50 minutes.

Kutner, N. G., R. Zhang, H.Barnhart, and A.J.Collins (2005). "Health status and quality of life reported by incident patients after 1 year on haemodialysis or peritoneal dialysis." Nephrology Dialysis Transplantation 20(10): 2159–2167.

Lamb, D. (1990). Organ Transplants and Ethics. London: Routledge.

Landsberg, A. (1995). Prosthetic memory: *Total Recall* and *Blade Runner*. *In* Cyperspace/Cyberbodies/Cyberpunk: Cultures of Technological Embodiment. M. Featherstone and R. Burrows, eds. Pp. 175–189. London: Sage Publications.

Lang, F. (1926). Metropolis. Germany, UFA: 153 minutes.

Lanza, A. M. (1971). The Incredible 2-Headed Transplant, U.S., Mutual General Corporartion/Trident Enterprises: 88 minutes.

Laporte, D. (2000 [1978]). History of Shit. Cambridge, MA: MIT Press.

Leach, E. (1967). Magical Hair: Myth and Cosmos. New York: Natural History Press.

Leder, D. (1990). The Absent Body. Chicago: University of Chicago Press.

Lerner, B. H. (2001). The Breast Cancer Wars: Hope, Fear, and the Pursuit of a Cure in Twentieth-Century America. New York: Oxford University Press.

Lingis, A. (1985). Libido: The French Existential Theories. Bloomington: Indiana University Press.

Lingis, A. (1994). Abuses. Berkeley and Los Angeles: University of California Press.

Lock, M. (2001). Twice Dead: Organ Transplants and the Reinvention of Death. Berkeley: University of California Press.

Lock, M. (2004). "Living cadavers and the calculation of death." Body & Society 10(2–3): 135–152.

Longmore, P. K. (1997). Conspicuous contribution and American cultural dilemmas: Telethon rituals of cleansing and renewal. *In* The Body and Physical Difference: Discourses of Disability. D. T. Mitchell and S. L. Snyder, eds. Pp. 134–158. Ann Arbor: University of Michigan Press.

Lorde, A. (1980). The Cancer Journals. San Francisco: Spinsters Ink.

Lossy, R. (1996). Time Pieces, A Collection of Poetry 1944–1996. Oakland, CA: RDR Books.

Loudon, J. B. (1977). On body products. *In* The Anthropology of the Body. J. Blacking, ed. Pp. 161–177. New York: Academic Press.

Lupton, D. (1995). The embodied computer/user. *In* Cyperspace/Cyberbodies/Cyberpunk: Cultures of Technological Embodiment. M. Featherstone and R. Burrows, eds. Pp. 97–112. London: Sage Publications.

MacCormack, C. P., ed. (1982). Ethnography of Fertility and Birth. New York: Academic Press.

MacLean, L. D., K. J. MacKinnon, and J.B.Dossetor (1971). Transplantation of the kidney: Human organ support and replacement. *In* Transplantation and Artificial Prostheses. J. D. Hardy, ed. Pp. 62–99. Springfield, IL: Charles C.Thomas.

Mairs, N. (1987). Plaintext: Deciphering a Woman's Life. New York: Perennial Library.

Mairs, N. (1996). Waist-high in the World. Boston: Beacon Press.

Makhmalbaf, M. (2001). Kandahar, Iran, Avatar: 85 minutes.

Malt, R. A. and C. F. McKhann (1964). "Replantation of severed arms." JAMA 189: 716.

Manderson, L., ed. (2005). Rethinking Wellbeing: Essays on Health, Disability and Disadvantage. Perth, Australia: Curtin University Press for API Network.

Manderson, L., E. Bennett, and S.Andajani-Sutjahjo (2006). "The social dynamics of the interview: Age, class and gender." Qualitative Health Research 16(10): 1317–1334.

Manderson, L. and S. Peake (2005). Men in motion: The performance of masculinity by disabled men. *In* Bodies in Commotion: Disability and Performance. P. Auslander and C. Sandahl, eds. Pp. 230–242. Ann Arbor: University of Michigan Press.

Manderson, L. and L. Stirling (2007). "The absent breast: Speaking of the mastectomied body." Feminism and Psychology 17(1): 75–92.

Manguel, A. (1996). A History of Reading. New York and London: Penguin Books.

Marcus, S. (1990 [1975]). Representations: Essays on Literature and Society. New York: Columbia University Press.

Matuschka. (2003). "Website." Retrieved April 10, 2003, from http://www.matuschka.net/matuschka.html.

Mauss, M. (1967). The Gift: Forms and Functions of Exchange in Archaic Societies. New York: W.W.Norton and Company, Inc.

Mendelssohn, D. C. (2004). "Empowerment of patient preference in dialysis modality selection." American Journal of Kidney Diseases 43(5): 930–932.

Merleau-Ponty, M. (1962). Phenomenology of Perception. London: Routledge and Kegan Paul.

Merleau-Ponty, M. (1968). The Visible and the Invisible. Chicago: Northwestern University Press.

Michelmore, K. (2001). "Transplant hand now amputated." The Sunday Age. Melbourne: 3.

Miner, M. (1997). Making up the stories as we go along: Men, women and narratives of disability. In The Body and Physical Difference: Discourses of Disability. D. T. Mitchell and S. L. Snyder, eds. Pp. 283–295. Ann Arbor: University of Michigan Press.

Mitchell, D.T. and S. L. Snyder (1997). Introduction: Disability studies and the double bind of representation. In The Body and Physical Difference: Discourses of Disability. D. T. Mitchell and S. L. Snyder, eds. Pp.1–34. Ann Arbor:University of Michigan Press.

Mitteness, L. S. and J. C. Barker (1995). "Stigmatizing a 'normal' condition: Urinary incontinence in late life." Medical Anthropology Quarterly 9(2): 188–210.

Moore, F. D. (1964). Give and Take – the Development of Tissue Transplantation. Philadelphia: WB Saunders.

Morgan, M. (2002). "The plumbing of modern life." Post-Colonial Studies Journal 5(2): 1–19.

Murphy, G. D. (2000). Race Against Time, U.S., TNT: 86 minutes.

Murphy, R. (1987). The Body Silent. London: Phoenix House.

Murray, C. J. (1996). Rethinking DALYs. In The Global Burden of Disease: A Comprehensive Assessment of Mortality and Disability from Diseases, Injuries and Risk Factors in 1990 and Projected to 2020. C. J. Murray and A. D. Lopez, eds. Pp. 1–98. Cambridge, MA: Harvard School of Population Health.

Murray, S. E. (n.d.). Painting as a spiritual journey: The works of Melissa Jane. Jakarta, Unpublished article distributed by the artist.

National Organization for Women (2004). "Tell Clear Channel, the FCC and Radio Stations to Stop "Breast Christmas Ever" Contest." NOW Action Alert.

Nelson, H. L. (1994). "The architect and the bee – Some reflections on postmortem pregnancy." Bioethics 8(3): 247–267.

Niccol, A. (1997). Gattaca, U.S., Columbia Pictures: 106 minutes.

Orwell, G. (1945). Animal Farm. London: Secker and Warburg.

Orwell, G. (1949). Nineteen Eighty-Four. London: Martin Secker & Warburg.

Panzarino, C. (1994). The Me in the Mirror. Seattle, WA: Seal Press.

Peake, S. and L. Manderson (2003). "The constraints of a normal life: The management of urinary incontinence by middle aged women." Women and Health 37(2): 37–51.

Peake, S., L. Manderson, and H.Potts (1999). "'Part and parcel of being a woman': Female urinary incontinence and constructions of control." Medical Anthropology Quarterly 13(3): 1–19.

Pernick, M. S. (1997). Defining the defective: Eugenics, aesthetics, and mass culture in early-twentieth-century America. *In* The Body and Physical Difference. Discourses of Disability. D. T. Mitchell and S. L. Snyder, eds. Pp. 89–110. Ann Arbor: University of Michigan Press.

Perry, J. E., L. R. Churchill, and H.S.Kirshner (2005). "The Terri Schiavo case: Legal, ethical, and medical perspectives." Annals of Internal Medicine 143(10): 744–748.

Piccinini, P. (2010). Beyond our kin, 2010. Press Release. Sydney, Roslyn Oxley9 Gallery. Retrieved June 2, 2011, from http://www.roslynoxley9.com.au/news/releases/2010/11/11/191/.

Piercy, M. (1976). Woman on the Edge of Time. New York: Alfred A. Knopf.

Pirani, C. (2002). "A great weight of hope in one pill." The Weekend Australian: 2.

Porter, J. I. (1997). Foreword. *In* The Body and Physical Difference. Discourses of Disability. D. T. Mitchell and S. L. Snyder, eds. Pp. xiii–xiv. Ann Arbor: University of Michigan Press.

Raz, H., ed. (1999). Living on the Margins: Women Writers on Breast Cancer. New York: Persea Books.

Red, E. (1991). Body Parts: 88 minutes.

Reitman, I. D. (1994). Junior, U.S.,Universal Pictures: 109 minutes.

Romei, S. (2001). "Mechanical heart man seriously ill." The Australian (August 15): 9.

Rosenbaum, M. E. and G. M. Roos (2000). Women's experiences of breast cancer. *In* Breast Cancer: Society Shapes an Epidemic. A. S. Kasper and S. J. Ferguson, eds. Pp. 153–181. New York: St. Martin's Press.

Rubin, H. A. and D. A. Shapiro (2005). Murderball, U.S., MTV Films: 88 minutes.

Russ, J. (1985 [1975]). The Female Man. London: Women's Press.

Sacks, O. W. (1984). A Leg to Stand On. New York: Harper and Row.

Sarbin, T. R. (1997). "The poetics of identity." Theory and Psychology 7: 67–82.

Scarry, E. (1985). The Body in Pain: The Making and Unmaking of the World. New York: Oxford University Press.

Scheibe, K. E. (2000). The Drama of Everyday Life. Cambridge, MA: Harvard University Press.

Scheper-Hughes, N. (2001). "Commodity fetishism in organs trafficking." Body and Society 7(2–3): 31–62.

Scheper-Hughes, N. (2002a). The global traffic in organs. *In* The Anthropology of Globalizaton. J. X. Inda and R. Rosaldo, eds. Pp. 270–310. London and Malden, MA: Basil Blackwell.

Scheper-Hughes, N. (2002b). Min(d)ing the body: On the trail of organ stealing rumors. *In* Exotic No More: Anthropology on the Front Lines. J. MacClancy, ed. Pp. 33–63. Chicago: University of Chicago Press.

Scheper-Hughes, N. (2004). "Parts unknown: Undercover ethnography of the organs-trafficking underworld." Ethnography 5: 29–73.

Schilder, P. (1950). The Image and Appearance of the Human Body : Studies in the Constructive Energies of the Psyche. New York: International Universities Press.

Schwarz, K. (1997). Missing the breast. Desire, disease and the singular effect of Amazons. *In* The Body in Parts: Fantasies of Corporeality in Early Modern Europe. D. Hillman and C. Mazzio, eds. Pp. 147–149. New York and London: Routledge.

Seymour, W. (1998). Remaking the Body: Rehabilitation and Change. Sydney: Allen and Unwin.

Sharp, L. A. A. (2006). Strange Harvest: Organ Transplants, Denatured Bodies, and the Transformed Self. Berkeley: University of California Press.

Sheard, S. and H. Power, eds. (2000). Body and City: Histories of Urban Public Health. Aldershot, UK: Ashgate.

Siegel, D. D. (1956). Invasion of the Body Snatchers, U.S., Allied Artists: 80 minutes.

Silverman, L. and D. Wishman (1970). The Amazing Transplant, U.S.: 80 minutes.

Simmons, R. G. and R. L. Simmons (1971). "Organ transplantation: A societal problem." Social Problems 19(1): 36–57.

Singelenberg, R. (1990). "The blood transfusion taboo of Jehovah's Witnesses: Origin, development and function of a controversial doctrine." Social Science and Medicine 31(4): 515–523.

Singer, P. (1994). Rethinking Life and Death: The Collapse of Our Traditional Values. New York: St. Martin's Press.

Sontag, S. (1978). Illness as Metaphor. London: Allen Lane.

Squier, S. M. (2004). Liminal Lives: Imagining the Human at the Frontiers of Biomedicine. Durham, NC: Duke University Press.

Stelarc (1996). Ping Body: Technical Information. Melton, Australia: Stelarc.

Stelarc (2002). "The extra ear, or an ear on an arm." Artlink. Australian Contemporary Art Quarterly 22(1): 9.

Stiker, H-J. (1999). A History of Disability. Ann Arbor: University of Michigan Press.

Stone, O. (1981). The Hand. U.S, Orion: 105 minutes.

Stone, O. (1989). Born on the Fourth of July. U.S., Universal: 145 minutes.

Straw, D. C. (2003). Home page. Office of Diabetes Association of Australia. Cottesloe, WA.

STV (1983). Taggart, Scottish Television.

Suskind, P. (1987 [1985]). Perfume: The Story of a Murderer. Harmondsworth, UK: Penguin.

Szreter, S. (1988). "The importance of social intervention in Britain's mortality decline c.1850-1914: A re-interpretation of the role of public health." Social History of Medicine 1(1): 1–37.

Taylor, R. M. (1997). "Reexamining the definition and criteria of death." Seminars in Neurology 17(3): 265–270.

Tempur-Pedic. (2002). "Home Page." Retrieved March 29, 2003, from http://www.tempurpedic.com/home.asp.

Thorpe, S. T. (1998). "The 'Grimm' Roots of Horror." Horror-Wood Webzine 2(13).

Transplant Society of Australia and New Zealand (2003). " General organ donor criteria. Guidelines for non-directed living renal donation in Australia." Retrieved May 6, 2007, from http://www.racp.edu.au/tsanz/oap7f.htm.

Urla, J. and J. Terry (1995). Introduction. In Deviant Bodies: Critical Perspectives on Difference in Science and Popular Culture. J. Terry and J. Urla, eds. Pp. 1–18. Bloomington: Indiana University Press.

Warin, M. (2003). "Miasmatic calories and saturating fats: Fear of contamination in anorexia." Culture, Medicine and Psychiatry 27(1): 77–93.

Warren, N. and L. Manderson (2008). "Constructing hope: Dis/continuity and narrative construction of recovery in the rehabilitation unit." Journal of Contemporary Ethnography 37(2): 180–201.

Warren, N., M. Markovic, and L. Manderson (2006). "Typologies of rural lay-health advocacy among rural women in Australia." Women and Health 43(4): 27–48.

Weiss, G. (1999). Body Images: Embodiment as Incorporeality. New York and London: Routledge.

Weldon, F. (1983). The Life and Loves of a She Devil. London: Hodder and Stoughton.

Whittaker, A., L. Manderson, and E. Cartwright (2010). "Patients beyond borders: A critical medical anthropology of medical travel." Medical Anthropology 29(4): 336–343.

Williams, G. R. (1971). Limp replantation. *In* Human Organ Support and Replacement: Transplantation and Artificial Prostheses. J. D. Hardy, ed. Pp. 415–430. Springfield, IL: Charles C. Thomas.

Wilson, R. R. (1995). Cyber(body)parts: Prosthetic consciousness. *In* Cyperspace/Cyberbodies/Cyberpunk: Cultures of Technological Embodiment. M. Featherstone and R. Burrows, eds. Pp. 239–259. London: Sage Publications.

Woo, J. (1997). Face/Off. U.S., Paramount Pictures: 138 minutes.

Wood, G. (2002). Living Dolls: A Magical History of the Quest for Mechanical Life. London: Faber and Faber.

Woodson, W. (2007). Nerve: Conversations with Lenore, U.S., Present Company Inc.: 29 minutes.

Wynn, B. (1971). Resurrection of Zachary Wheeler. U.S., Vidtronics: 100 minutes.

Yang, Y. G. and M. Sykes (2007). "Tolerance in xenotransplantation." Current Opinion in Organ Transplantation 12(2): 169–175.

Young, I.M. (1990). Breasted experience: The look and the feeling." *In* Throwing Like a Girl and Other Essays in Feminist Philosophy and Social Theory. I.M. Young, ed. Pp.189–209. Bloomington: Indiana University Press.

Zola, I. K. (1982). Missing Pieces: A Chronicle of Living with a Disability. Philadelphia: Temple University Press.

Zurbarán, F. d. (1630–1633). St. Agatha. Montpellier, France: Musée Fabre.

Index 🙖

Page numbers in **boldface** refer to figures.

Gosling, Ju, 42, 43, **43**, 86–89, **88**, 264
Grealy, Lucy, 74–75, 258

Habitus, 28, 52, 94, 96, 97, 102, 106
Hand, The, 82
Hand of Orlac, The, 81, **82**, 83, 238
Haraway, Donna, 58
Health advocacy, 173, **174**, 179, 202, 205
Hearing aids, 63–64, 252, 255
    bionic ear, 64
    cochlear implant, 64–65
Hoghe, Raimund, 89, 201
Humor, 118, 232–233, 238

Incontinence, 125–126, 137–139
    in women, 36–37, 137, 150, 155
Identity, 72
    building, 67
If, 79
Independence, 101, 118, 122, 124, 126
    loss of, 161–162
Industrial design, 69–70, 131, 251, 252–254
Industrialized settings, 30, 36, 37, 59, 60, 67, 75, 95, 140, 211, 245,
Industrialization, 78
Inequality, 34, 60, 67, 69, 90, 91, 95, 262
    and race, 238
    see also gender
Intimacy, *see* sexual intimacy
Invasion of the Body Snatchers, The, 77

Jackson, Cindy, 76
John Q, 250–251, **250**
Johnson, Susan, 134
Jones, Sharon, 178, **180–181**, 206 n. 2
Junior, 251

Kandahar, 95
Kidney organs, **227**
    and cadaver, 225
    and family, 218–225
    and grief, 228–230
    and non-directed living donation, 230–231

❧ About the Author

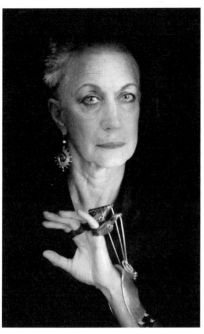

Photograph by Sarah Walker; 2011.

Lenore Manderson is an inaugural Australian Research Council Federation Fellow and Professor of Medical Anthropology in the Faculty of Medicine, Nursing and Health Sciences, and the Faculty of Arts, at Monash University, in Melbourne, Australia. As a medical anthropologist, public health scholar and social historian of medicine, she has been active in education and research on inequality, social exclusion and marginality, infectious and chronic disease, gender and sexuality, in Australia, Southeast and East Asia, and Africa. She has published over 500 works, including the co-edited volumes *Global Health Policy, Local Realities* (2000), *Social Capital and Social Justice* (2009), and *Chronic Conditions, Fluid States* (2010). She collaborated in and is the subject of the film, *Nerve* (USA, 2007). She is a Fellow of the Academy of Social Sciences in Australia and the World Academy of Art and Science, and is Editor of the international journal *Medical Anthropology*.